Directing Research in Primary Care

David A. Katerndahl, MD, MA

T0143293

Radcliffe Publishing
Oxford • Seattle

Radcliffe Publishing Ltd
18 Marcham Road
Abingdon
Oxon OX14 1AA
United Kingdom

www.radcliffe-oxford.com
Electronic catalogue and worldwide online ordering facility.

British Library Cataloguing in Publication Data

A catalogue record for this book is available from the British Library.

ISBN-10 1 84619 028 2
ISBN-13 978 1 84619 028 5

Typeset by Anne Joshua & Associates, Oxford, UK
Printed and bound by TJ International Ltd, Padstow, Cornwall, UK

Contents

Preface

Why This Book; Why Now?

With a meager 20- to 30-year tradition of research output in primary care, why is a guidebook describing the development of a departmental research program needed? The answer is that recent developments and anticipated future developments suggest that things are changing, that the recognition of and need for primary care research may have turned a corner in academic circles. First, within primary care disciplines, the perception of research has changed. Evidence-based medicine is increasingly embraced. Organizations such as the American Academy of Family Physicians are investing in research development and trying to change the negative perceptions of research held by its members. A new research journal, the *Annals of Family Medicine*, was successfully launched by a consortium of primary care groups. The membership of the North American Primary Care Research Group has grown from 492 in 1997 to 853 in 2003. Second, outside of primary care, the perception of our research has changed. Although the funding of the Agency for Healthcare Research and Quality is still inadequate, other National Institutes of Health (NIH) institutes recognize the need for research in primary care settings, are beginning to fund studies involving practice-based research networks, and actively seek participation of primary care researchers on their study sections. Finally, potential future development will rely heavily upon a primary care base, thus needing a strong research base. Such developments include national healthcare reform that can only succeed through a primary care foundation, growing concern about health disparities among certain segments of the population (segments which depend upon primary care for their access to healthcare services), and national initiatives to improve the quality of care while reducing medical errors (necessitating a focus on primary care co-ordination of services in our complex system). The Future of Family Medicine Project clearly links the need for research to such reforms.

How will the Development of Departmental Research be Approached?

Section I focuses on the research environment outside of the primary care department or division and the roles administrators play in forming that environment. After reviewing the current primary care and family medicine research environments, the section looks at the standards, environment, and attitudes that constitute the ingredients of the research environment, and reviews the roles that the dean, the department chair, the individual researcher, and the research director have in providing a research environment that is conducive to primary care research. Finally, the section focuses upon the responsibilities of the research director. Section II deals with developing individual researchers, from motivating the faculty to get involved in research, to the characteristics of productive researchers. The section describes strategies for the development of researchers, including preparing for promotion and planning their careers. Section III deals with development of research from a departmental standpoint, looking at the qualities of productive departments as well as developmental stages and plans. The section concludes with a discussion of evaluating the success of such development. Section IV changes from the traditional perspective of investigator and departmental development, to viewing building research capacity from the framework of complexity science. After presenting evidence that research units are in fact complex adaptive systems, the section discusses how building research capacity would differ from traditional approaches if done from a complexity science perspective. Finally, Section V reviews recent developments that are important to the future development of primary care research, and presents recommendations designed to foster a positive environment for future primary care researchers.

What is Unique About This Book?

Perhaps nothing; perhaps everything. Each chapter begins with a brief vignette. If you see yourself or a colleague within that vignette, that chapter is likely to "speak to you". The body of each chapter is an amalgam of personal experience in capacity building at the national, state, and local level, along with a review of the literature. Finally, each chapter ends with a synthesis to give you the high points and attempt to resolve any contradictions presented. Thus, this book is also unique in its devotion to building research capacity at both the micro- and macro-levels, the individual, and departmental levels. Finally, this book attempts to present capacity building not only from the traditional approach, but from a complexity science approach as well.

Who Should Read This Book?

Although written from the perspective of the director of research within an academic primary care department or division (or someone considering such a position), others may benefit from this manuscript. Medical deans seeking to provide an academic environment conducive to primary care and interdisciplinary research should find this book helpful. Individual primary care researchers will benefit personally from the advice presented in Section II, but may also find the larger perspective discussed in the other sections helpful in understanding their position within the greater context. Finally, the departmental chair who wants to develop or support research within his or her department will benefit from the description of what is needed for such development, its realistic timeline, and the qualities needed in its research director. I hope everyone – researcher, administrator, and scholar – can take something from the time spent in reading these pages.

David A. Katerndahl, MD, MA
Professor
Department of Family and Community Medicine
University of Texas Health Science Center at San Antonio
San Antonio, Texas
November 2005

About the Author

David Katerndahl has long been committed to building research capacity in primary care. After receiving his medical degree from the University of Illinois and completing a family medicine residency at Ohio State University, he completed a fellowship at Ohio State University and received a masters' degree in education. After three years in private practice in rural Illinois, he joined the faculty in the Department of Family and Community Medicine at the University of Texas Health Science Center at San Antonio in 1984.

In addition to serving as Director of Research in the Department of Family and Community Medicine, he has been active in research development through the Texas Academy of Family Physicians, serving as chairs of its Research Committee and the Research Grants Committee for its foundation. At an international level, Dr Katerndahl has served on the North American Primary Care Research Group's (NAPCRG's) Committee for Building Research Capacity, founding the successful Grant Generating Project and conducting a series of research career planning workshops, and as co-chair of the Qualitative/Quantitative Methodology and Complexity Science Special Interest Groups. In addition, he founded and co-co-ordinated the annual Primary Care Research Methods and Statistics Conference, now in its 20th year. Finally, he has authored or co-authored 17 articles and editorials on building research capacity within primary care. For his efforts in promoting research development, Dr Katerndahl was awarded the Presidential Award of Merit in 2004 by the Texas Academy of Family Physicians, and the President's Recognition Award in 2002 by the North American Primary Care Research Group.

Acknowledgments

I wish to thank my colleagues in the Department of Family and Community Medicine at the University of Texas Health Science Center in San Antonio for their ongoing support, their tolerance of evaluation activities, and their willingness to serve as academic "guinea pigs". I appreciate the selfless input and commitment of Benjamin Crabtree and Reuben McDaniel, and numerous primary care researchers in the North American Primary Care Research Group. Finally, I wish to express my personal gratitude to Robert Ferrer and Sandra Burge for their thoughtful critique of this manuscript.

Abbreviations

AAFP	American Academy of Family Physicians
AAU	Academic Administrative Unit
AFMO	Academic Family Medicine Organizations
AHCPR	Agency for Health Care Policy and Research
AHRQ	Agency for Healthcare Research and Quality
AMA	American Medical Association
AOA	Alpha Omega Alpha
ASPN	Ambulatory Sentinel Practice Network
CME	continuing medical education
COV	coefficient of variation
CV	curriculum vitae
DHHS	Department of Health and Human Services
FARES	Faculty Activities and Research Environment Survey
FFM	Future of Family Medicine
FPIN	Family Practice Inquiries Network
HEENT	head, eyes, ears, nose, and throat
HIPAA	Health Insurance Portability and Accountability Act
HRSA	Health Resources and Services Administration
ICPC	International Classification of Primary Care
IRB	Institutional Review Board
M&O	maintenance and operations
NAPCRG	North American Primary Care Research Group
NIH	National Institutes of Health
NRSA	National Research Service Award
OGM	Office of Grants Management
OR	odds ratio
P&T	promotion and tenure
PBRNs	practice-based research networks
PHS	Public Health Service
POEM	patient-oriented evidence that matters
RFA	Request for Applications
RWJ	Robert Wood Johnson
SCI	Science Citation Index
SSCI	Social Science Citation Index
STFM	Society of Teachers of Family Medicine
SWOG	South West Oncology Group
TQM	total quality management

I wish to dedicate this book to Mitzie, Tiffany, Tarah, and Jenny for their patience and understanding during my numerous absences at meetings, my ill-tempered periods of grant writing, and my hours of writing seclusion. Whatever I may accomplish professionally is only possible through your loving support.

Section I

Directing Research

## Chapter 1

The Primary Care Research Environment

Vignette

Fresh from her clinical rotations, A.Z. was in a quandary, pressured to begin the hunt for a residency program but uncertain about what discipline to choose. Enjoying all of her basic clerkships, she was leaning towards family medicine but she was concerned about its future. What appealed to her was the emphasis on patient care and the commitment to long-term relationships with patients, as well as the focus on teaching among its faculty. It seemed the natural choice for someone who was "sick" of hearing about the latest obscure study among tertiary care patients published in the *New England Journal of Medicine*, someone who just wanted to care for patients and their families. She actually liked the idea of belonging to the "counterculture" of family medicine, committed to everything that the subspecialists held in low esteem. She had been a "rebel" in college and the role suited her, but now family medicine was calling for a "culture of inquiry" committed to primary care research. It seemed as though the counterculture was selling out; that could not bode well for the discipline.

Primary care research is essentially ignored in "ivory tower" medicine. But its infancy is not surprising. Family medicine became a specialty in 1969; general internal medicine and ambulatory pediatrics are even younger. Their research structures are naturally less well established than those of specialty medicine. Consequently, primary care research does not have the tradition or acceptance of the rest of the clinical research establishment.

Yet, the trends in American medicine and healthcare are towards ambulatory care, preventive medicine, cost containment, and healthcare delivery . . . and primary care that will provide for these needs. Hence, research in these areas is most appropriately done by the primary care disciplines themselves. Recently, even the National Institutes of Health are devoting attention to primary care research. It is only proper that the funds appropriated for primary care research be utilized by the primary care disciplines for conducting research within their arena of practice.

Primary care must assume its role in the menagerie of clinical research. Although basic research has been essential to all of the major breakthroughs in medicine, it is clinical research that applies the basic knowledge to the patient. Generally, clinical research takes the small laboratory-based bits of new information and synthesizes them into a practical patient-based reality. This translation process has contributed so much to the relative explosion of medical knowledge over the past 30–40 years. Primary care research takes this translation process one step further by applying the findings of tertiary care clinical research to the primary care setting. In addition, primary care research is unique in its focus on the natural history of common problems, the non-medical influences on health, and effective models of care. Hence, primary care research represents the ultimate in the synthesis–application process of clinical research.

The Primary Care Research Environment

A "profession" is distinguished from a "trade" by its effort to seek new knowledge to better serve mankind and contribute to the body of general knowledge (Bawden, 1983). The value of research to the primary care physician is manifold. Research helps to establish a discipline and generate new knowledge; primary care research also seeks to provide information in areas previously ignored, thus improving healthcare. In addition, research makes us more critical, improving critical appraisal skills, and thereby improving our teaching and relationships with other disciplines (Curtis, 1980).

In general, for primary care to realistically conduct high-quality research in sufficient quantities to make a difference, the research environment must include certain resources (i.e. research tools, library access), interchange (i.e. collabora-tors, consultants, collegial stimulation), forums for communication of results, and involvement of practice settings (Geyman, 1978). When primary care research began, it faced numerous obstacles. In addition to a lack of researchers and research journals, personal obstacles such as lack of confidence and an unwill-ingness to study ourselves, coupled with the demands of clinical service held us back (Colton, 1980). Even after the pioneers took the lead, primary care research progressed slowly, mired in a sea of conflicting priorities. Unrealistic demands were placed on researchers, who were expected to continue heavy teaching and administrative loads at the expense of research time. Inadequate resources (researchers, space, equipment, funding) continued to plague our efforts. Researchers themselves were also part of the problem, possessing negative attitudes concerning research and lacking commitment. Ultimately, the lack of progress reflected apathy from leaders and the lack of a research tradition (Copp, 1984; Huth, 1986). As late as 1996, primary care research continued to battle against the same barriers. There were problems with investigators (lack of a critical mass, competing demands), the environment (lack of mentors, no research culture), research ideas (reductionism approach, lack of theory), methods (study design and measurement problems, access to populations), and funding.

However, efforts were put in place to attack each of these barriers. The lack of investigators led to the development of "incubator" environments and training opportunities. Limitations of the research environment led investigators to develop collaborations and utilize multiple mentors. Movements led us to promote the primary care perspective on research issues and to develop theoret-ical underpinnings. Problems with reductionist methods and "heavily selected" populations led researchers to develop and adapt new methods, emphasizing multimethod approaches and the formation of research laboratories. Finally, the lack of research funding caused primary care leaders to push for federal support (such as the Agency for Healthcare Research and Quality (AHRQ)) and investigators to seek alternative funding sources such as foundations and managed care organizations, while also attempting to link primary care studies to initiatives in specialist institutes (Stange, 1996).

In 1993, the Agency for Healthcare Research and Quality (then the Agency for Health Care Policy and Research) developed a set of recommendations to promote primary care research; at a national level, the Department of Health and Human Services (DHHS) and the Public Health Service (PHS) should increase their support for primary care research, and AHRQ would develop a research agenda. These institutions should also develop their own unique strategies. Hence, while PHS supported the development of leadership skills in researchers, AHRQ would support the development of practice-based research networks (PBRNs) and of research infrastructure within primary care departments. In addition, AHRQ would promote the development of linkages between disciplines and researchers. At the individual level, AHRQ emphasized the need for primary care research fellowships, and supported career development of researchers and technical support for grant proposals. Finally, PHS would support efforts to teach research skills to medical students (Agency for Health Care Policy and Research (AHCPR), 1993). Despite the recognition of the barriers and opportunities mentioned above, and the support of AHRQ and PHS, the research environment for primary care is still less than optimal. But is the research environment in family medicine any better?

The Family Practice Research Environment

Although research is recognized as critical to defining the discipline of family medicine (Taylor, 1990), to ensuring that family physicians do not provide out-of-date therapy (Antman *et al*, 1992), and to attracting qualified medical students into the discipline (Bowman *et al*, 1996), the family practice environment is not supportive of research because family practitioners do not value research. Even though family physicians frequently ask clinical questions and seek answers (Gorman and Helfand, 1995), they rarely use research sources. Family physicians rate research as poorer than all other information sources in terms of understandability and applicability. In addition, research is rated as more credible than only one other source – pharmaceutical representatives (Connelly *et al.* 1990). Consequently, family physicians rarely use research articles as sources of information, preferring to use colleagues and textbooks (Verhoeven *et al*, 1995). When offered free copies of the *Archives of Family Medicine*, only 19 000 of the 100 000 eligible physicians actually requested the journal. These negative attitudes towards research are reflected in the poor attendance by practitioners at research meetings and in the fate of its journals. Although the *American Family Physician* with its review article format enjoys success, family medicine research journals have struggled. The *Family Practice Research Journal* and *Archives of Family Medicine* have terminated publication due to the lack of subscriptions by practitioners, the resultant lack of advertisement dollars, and consequently financial collapse.

Do other specialties or other primary care disciplines share these attitudes? Compared with other specialties, family medicine is less likely to require research to be conducted by its residents (Blake *et al*, 1994; Temte *et al*, 1994; Taniguchi and Johnson, 1994; DeHaven *et al*, 1997). Compared with other primary care specialties, family medicine also lags behind. This lack of research emphasis is true in terms of the use of research (Connelly *et al*, 1990), research requirements during residency training (Alguire *et al*, 1996), and the availability of research fellowships (Elward *et al*, 1994; Rodnick, 1999). Thus, research values differ among primary care disciplines. However, family physicians in other countries do not share these attitudes. English family physicians use refereed journals more often (Prescott *et al*, 1997). In addition, Danish family physicians accept the need for involvement in research (Almind, 1993) and 62% of English family practices are actually involved in research (Kenkre *et al*, 1993). Thus, negative attitudes towards research may be unique to American family physicians.

If the research environment in the discipline of American family medicine is not supportive of research, is the environment any more supportive for departments of family medicine within academic health centers?

The Academic Research Environment

Academic Health Centers

Many faculties at academic health centers feel that there has been an increase in institutional support for clinical research in the past five years. This is true of administrative support, patient and staff recruitment, and overall investment. However, the greatest perceived gains have been in the area of clinical trials rather than in more traditional primary care areas, such as outcomes research and translational research. In addition, despite the perceived increased institutional support for research, these faculties generally feel that clinical research is not the institution's top priority (Oinonen *et al*, 2001).

In fact, a recent survey of department chairs and research administrators suggests that they are less optimistic about the future of clinical research at academic health centers. Generally, they felt that the environment for clinical research was less healthy than it had been in the past, and that clinical researchers face increasing challenges due to decreasing revenues, limited funding, increased time commitments to practice, and changes in review procedures of institutional review boards (Campbell *et al*, 2001).

This may be particularly true for primary care research. In 1986, 26% of general internists felt that one of the reasons for inadequate research in primary care was the denigration they experienced from subspecialists (Huth, 1986). Ten years later, primary care research is still held in low regard by specialists in academic health centers. Not only do subspecialist faculties rate the quality of primary care research lower than do primary care faculties, but department chairs and research directors rate it lower than do faculties (Block *et al*, 1996).

All clinical researchers in academic health centers face significant challenges, but primary care researchers in these centers face more challenges than do other investigators. The research environment within primary care in these academic centers is even more tenuous.

Departments/Divisions of Primary Care

The opportunity for research is a significant motivational factor in the decision for primary care physicians to enter academic medicine (Hueston, 1993a). Yet, few primary care faculty members spend significant amounts of time committed to research. Part of the reason rests with the limitations placed on primary care research at the levels of the academic health center and the discipline. However, the supportiveness of the department is also critical and can often offset pressures at higher levels.

Unfortunately, departmental environments often do not support research. A critical person in the perceived support for research is the departmental chair. In 1994, family medicine chairs ranked the importance of research, non-research scholarship, and fellowship as seventh, eighth, and ninth out of nine areas (Katerndahl, 1994). This lack of support for scholarship may reflect the lack of research experience among chairs. As of 1992, fewer than 20% of chairs had research experience. Although younger chairs reported more research training and skills than did their older counterparts, they had no more experience in conducting research (Murata *et al*, 1992). And the proportion of chairs with research experience has not increased much since then. Thus, a lack of research experience may lead to a perception that research is less important or vice versa. In either case, the perception that research is of less importance than patient care or teaching, for example, will probably translate into a less supportive departmental environment for research.

Whence We Came

New research is built upon the foundations of past research. Each new study adds to the tradition of medical research. In order to understand where we need to go, we need to first know where we have been. Evaluating the current status of medical research is difficult because not all good research is published and not all published research is good. Indeed, it is appropriate at times to do research with no intention of publishing. However, the only practical way to assess the status of primary care research is to assess the status of the medical literature in general.

By sheer volume alone, the medical literature is impressive. The rate of its growth is staggering. The 20,000 biomedical journals disseminate this information at an expanding rate of 6–7% each year, doubling every 10–15 years. For example, in a 10-year period, there were 16,000 citations on "viral hepatitis"! Keeping up with this explosion would require you to read 200 articles per month just to keep up with the 10 leading medical journals. To keep up with every advance would require you to read about 40,000 articles each week (Price, 1963). However, it appears that North American physicians spend between three hours per week and 5.5 hours per month reading journals (Haynes *et al*, 1986). Biomedical knowledge is expanding at a truly awesome rate.

Activity

In 1990, few family physicians or general pediatrics faculty considered themselves primarily to be researchers (American Medical Association (AMA), 1988; Brotherton *et al*, 1997). Even in 1993, only about 10% of faculty time in university-based and university-administered programs was spent on research (Hueston, 1993a). This is consistent with the state of support for research in family medicine as presented in 1983. Of the 749 family practice programs surveyed, only 37% had a visible research program, and only 54% had a research co-ordinator.

Although over 70% of programs offered assistance with study design, writing, computer programming, and analysis, only 45% had research assistants available. In fact, more than half of the programs reported less than 10% of faculty time for research (Culpepper and Franks, 1983). These figures are similar to the support available to allied health faculty reported in 1993 (Peterson *et al*, 1993) and the research time availability is similar to that reported for both allied health faculty and perfusion faculty in 1987 and 1993 (Bennett and Beckley, 1987; Peterson *et al*, 1993). Although these figures agree with the observation that from 1980 to 1989 the proportion of articles from practitioners in the *British Journal of General Practice* dropped (Pitts, 1991), they differ from a survey that indicated that 62% of general practices were involved in research in 1993 (Kenkre *et al*, 1993).

Quality

Study designs used in papers in the family medicine literature have been less sophisticated than those of the general medical literature. Between 1977 and 1979, fewer than 10% of articles published in the *Journal of Family Practice* and the *Journal of the Royal College of General Practice* used retrospective, cohort, and clinical trial designs (Frey and Frey, 1981). A study of papers published in *Family Medicine* found that 32% were case reports. In the study of the *Journal of Family Practice* from 1974 to 1983, almost 90% of papers used a cross-sectional design (Geyman and Berg, 1984), similar to general practice research in New Zealand (Richards, 1980). Over a 5-year period, observational research papers increased, while reviews decreased. Experimental research remained steady at a low level (Geyman and Berg, 1984). However, from 1984 to 1988, both descriptive and experimental research in the *Journal of Family Practice* increased (Geyman and Berg, 1989). However, a review of North American Primary Care Research Group (NAPCRG) abstracts from 1977 to 1987 found that cross-sectional research was presented 58% of the time with prospective and experimental research accounting for 15% each of the remainder (Muncie *et al*, 1990). Even though published clinical trials increased in the US literature from 1987 to 1991 (Silagy *et al*, 1994), the proportion of Australian clinical trials as reported in 1992 was still only 15%, with descriptive research accounting for 52% (Silagy *et al*, 1992). This appears to be in contradiction to the heavy involvement of general practices in clinical trials as reported in the United Kingdom, where 68% of practices reported being involved in a therapeutic trial (Kenkre *et al*, 1993). In fact, compared with a sample of articles published in *JAMA* and the *New England Journal of Medicine* in 1989, articles published in US family medicine journals used similar research designs (Marvel *et al*, 1991). However, in a survey of publications by family medicine researchers in 2000, cross-sectional designs still predominated (56%) with cohort (18%) and randomized trials (12%) accounting for similar proportions to those found in 1990 (Merenstein *et al*, 2003).

   Other than via study design, quality in research is a matter of judgment and is therefore difficult to assess. Although most publications in the *Journal of General Internal Medicine* were felt to be acceptable, several problem areas were reported in 1989. These included generalizability, informed consent, reliability assessment, and use of statistics (Cooper and Zangwill, 1989). In addition, two studies have addressed the quality of clinical trials reported in the family medicine literature. On the one hand, Silagy and Jewell (1994) found that, over the 39 years of trials published in the *British Journal of General Practice*, there was a trend towards decreasing control of bias, but while Sonis and Joines (1994) agreed that the quality of the trials published from 1974 to 1991 in the *Journal of Family Practice* was poor, they also found that the quality was increasing over the years.

The relevance of research to practice is also a measure of quality. Once Curry and MacIntyre (1982) established the concordance of family practice diagnostic content across 15 studies, it became possible to assess the agreement between these rankings and the content of the family medicine literature. Katerndahl *et al* (1998) found significant correlations ($r_s = 0.66$ and $r_s = 0.78$) between the ranked contents of practice and family medicine research from 1990 to 1996. Those topics that were over-represented in the research literature tended to be either preventive (i.e. alcohol use, contraception, dyslipidemia) or life-threatening (i.e. cancer, violence, AIDS) in nature. When the family medicine research publications of 2000 were evaluated, 46% were found to be relevant. In fact, 26% were felt to be highly relevant. On the other hand, of the 170 publications reviewed, only 22 (13%) were both highly relevant and valid, suggestive of patient-oriented evidence that matters (POEMs) (Merenstein *et al*, 2003). POEMs are summaries of research studies that address questions frequently seen by primary care physicians, that report outcomes considered important by physicians and patients, and that have the potential to change physician behavior.

Publication Patterns

How productive are primary care researchers? Between 1990 and 1996, Katerndahl *et al* (1998) found that family medicine researchers published over 1200 research studies. Based upon articles published in MEDLINE-included sources, Table 1.1 summarizes the quantity of research publications between 1990 and 1996. Such figures are probably compatible with those of Weiss (2002) who found that Society of Teachers of Family Medicine (STFM) members published 749 research and non-research articles in 1989, 1040 in 1994, and 669 in 1999. Pathman *et al* (2002) found that family medicine researchers published 484 research studies in 1999 and 496 in 2000 not limited to MEDLINE-based journals; twice as many as those found by Katerndahl *et al* (1998). Using different methods of assessment, these studies confirm the lack of steady growth (and possibly even decline) in research publications over time. However, in 2003, family medicine researchers published 765 research articles (Pathman *et al*, 2005). Marchiori *et al* (1998) reported that, whereas medicine faculty published between 2.0 and 2.2 articles per faculty member per year on average, general internal medicine faculty published 1.8 articles. Other ''primary care'' faculty researchers published even less with nursing faculties averaging 0.7 publications and chiropractic faculties averaging only 0.3 publications per researcher. Although the mean number of publications per family medicine researcher was 2.24 for 1999–2000, the majority of researchers had only one publication during that time; only 8% had over five research publications (Pathman *et al*, 2002). Even though the total number of research articles increased in 2003, the average number per researcher dropped to 1.89 articles per researcher (Pathman *et al*, 2005). This is consistent with the findings of Weiss (2002) that only 8.5% of STFM members published more than one article in 1999; down from 16% in both 1989 and 1994. These studies suggest that, although the discipline produces a significant body of literature, its growth rate is declining. This decline is despite the observation that 48% of STFM and NAPCRG presentations result in publication within five years (Elder and Blake, 1994). A similar drop in research publications was seen among productive science education researchers from 1980–1984 to 1990–1994 (Barrow, 2002), suggesting that such a drop among productive researchers may be a normal development. A 2000 survey of family medicine faculty found that only 48% had submitted a manuscript for publication during the previous two years; overall, the mean numbers of manuscripts submitted and accepted for publication were 1.20 and 0.95 during this period (Brocato and Mavis, 2005).

Table 1.1 Family Medicine Research Publications in MEDLINE-based Journals from 1990 to 1996

Measure	1990	1992	1994	1996
Total number of research publications	125	300	140	290
Percentage in family medicine journals	55	53	49	80

Just as 19% of articles published in family medicine journals originate from other disciplines (Wagner *et al*, 1994), primary care researchers publish in non-primary care journals as well. Ingram (1992) found that half of all family medicine publications appeared in non-family medicine journals in both 1979 and 1989. Weiss (2002) found that of all the articles published in 1989, 1994, and 1999 by STFM members, only 12% were published in the *Journal of Family Practice* and 11% were published in *Family Medicine*. Similarly, Elder and Blake (1994) found that 44% of publications originating as STFM or NAPCRG presentations appeared in non-family medicine journals. In fact, Katerndahl *et al* (1998) determined that, between 1990 and 1996, 41% of research publications involving family medicine researchers appeared in non-family medicine journals. Most recently, Merenstein *et al* (2003) found that 42% of family medicine research publications appeared in non-family medicine journals. But these figures are not unique to family medicine; for example, 49% of rheumatology research articles were published in non-rheumatology journals (Ramos-Remus *et al*, 1993). Finally, Pathman *et al* (2002) found that, of the 980 research articles published in 1999 and 2000 by family medicine researchers, 31% appeared in three family medicine journals out of the 236 journals in which family medicine research was published; 30 articles were published in top general medicine journals – *JAMA*, *New England Journal of Medicine*, *British Medical Journal*, and *Annals of Internal Medicine*. However, family medicine researchers are generally not publishing in non-family medicine journals due to lack of space, but rather for other reasons, including wider readership (79%) and more prestige (28%) (Weiss, 1990). The drop in science education research publications found by Barrow (2002) was primarily seen in science education's top journal, suggesting that these productive researchers may have switched to publishing outside of their discipline.

Synthesis

Hence, although inroads have been made over the past two decades, the research environment in primary care is still tenuous. Increased pressures on academic centers may make their research environments less supportive than they were previously. Finally, the lack of recognition of the importance of research by departmental chairs does not bode well for the support within departments.

Although based upon studies frequently more than a decade old, this review suggests that the general medical literature may be expanding at an impressive rate, but has suffered from a lack of methodological quality and sophistication. Such observations are mirrored in the primary care literature as well. Although quality and sophistication are improving in general, such trends in primary care have lagged behind those in the general medical literature. Of particular concern is the evidence that research productivity in primary care may be declining, and that those articles that are published are appearing in non-primary care journals. Clearly, more recent research in this area is needed.

To medical deans, primary care department or division chairs, or directors of research, this chapter suggests the difficulty that lies ahead. It also suggests the challenges facing the primary care investigator in the current medical climate. These difficulties are particularly important if you, as director of research, are tasked with starting a program where none exists. Conducting research within this non-supportive reality is a challenge. What are the issues inherent in conducting primary care research and who is responsible for the research standards, environment, and attitudes involved? What can the leadership working within such environments do to mitigate these limitations and facilitate research among faculty?

## Chapter 2

The Big Picture

Vignette

This was not how primary care faculty should treat one another! B.Y. had been pursuing a research career for three years now in a department known for its research. He felt that he had been a "good citizen", helping others on their projects while inviting their involvement on his. But after all of his work, a more senior faculty member had submitted the manuscript without including him as a co-author. And no one else was supporting him in this matter. It made him think twice about presenting his ideas for a new study to the other faculty for their comments at the departmental research meeting. How could he be certain that one of them wouldn't submit a grant using his design before he could? For that matter, could he even share his ideas at the STFM meeting without running the risk of being exploited?

Much of the body of knowledge in primary care is drawn from the research of others on tertiary care patients. This is not acceptable and may be very misleading, because such research is conducted on highly selected patients, not representative of those seen in primary care settings. New knowledge is needed because current knowledge is incomplete and because we face new challenges.

Defining the Discipline

McWhinney (1966) stated that there are four criteria for a "discipline". They include:

1. a unique field of action
2. a defined body of knowledge
3. active research
4. intellectually rigorous training.

Although the boundaries are sometimes obscured, primary care has a unique field of action. Primary care research should focus within this unique field of action.

New knowledge is needed to define the discipline. Tacit knowledge must be made explicit and we must seek to optimize our roles as family physicians if the healthcare system is to survive (Stange *et al*, 2001). Such research should address the full gambit of human experience from the personal to the impersonal, from the microscopic to the macroscopic. Figure 2.1 describes the scope of primary care research from the level of research focus to the level of experience, and the methods for investigating each. This framework emphasizes the vastness of scope relevant to primary care as well as the generalizability of its results. Primary care research is not just about the disease focus of specialty research, but is also about family-focused investigation and health services research. This framework can structure the primary care knowledge base and recognizes the need for integration between personal and impersonal experience (Stange *et al*, 2001).

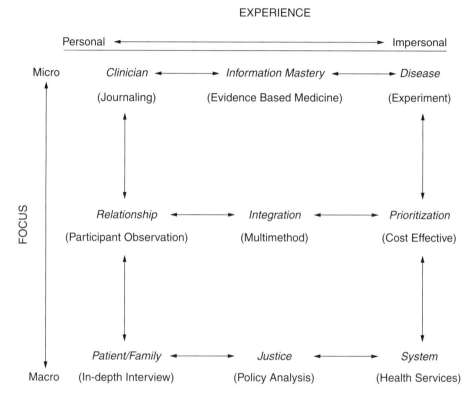

Figure 2.1 Scope of Primary Care Research (Stange *et al*, 2001). Reprinted with permission from the Society of Teachers of Family Medicine, www.stfm.org.

Only through high-quality research on primary care patients conducted by researchers who understand primary care can such a defined body of knowledge be established. On the one hand, research is needed on the content of primary care, including the characteristics of primary care, common illnesses and presentations, and the natural history of disease. On the other hand, primary care research should address particular aspects of the delivery of healthcare, and include cross-cultural studies and studies on environmental, occupational, and community health. In addition, primary care research must address family aspects of health, such as family epidemiology, and the effects of family and community on illness patterns (Perkoff, 1981).

Although research activity within primary care is underway and may be more extensive than we realize, it is far from adequate. There are several reasons for this lack of research activity, which we will address in more detail later in this book. However, one reason is the lack of intellectually rigorous training in many departments and residency programs. This book is intended to help in establishing and nurturing such training.

Research Ingredients

The climate for research in primary care is defined by its research standards, its environment, and the personal attitudes of its members (Geyman, 1978). Although responsibility for each is often shared, in reality, research standards are set by the discipline, environment is determined locally by the department or residency program, and attitudes are set by the individual researchers.

Standards

When we talk about standards and norms, we are talking about ethical standards and research norms. The recent implementation of Health Insurance Portability and Accountability Act (HIPAA) requirements has placed a new level of ethical burden upon researchers in terms of access of records and informed consent. Although we can set personal standards, it should ultimately be the discipline that sets the ethical standards for its research. A survey of clinical scientists and administrators found that all of them felt that falsification of data and plagiarism were unethical, and most (> 85%) felt that deliberately misleading readers was unethical. However, less than 85% considered sloppy research methods and conflict of interests as unethical (Korenman *et al*, 1998). Such discipline-wide beliefs set the ethical standards for research in a discipline.

Emanuel *et al* (2000) proposed seven characteristics for ethical research. The study must have value by potentially enhancing health or knowledge. The study must be rigorous, having scientific validity. Subject selection must also be fair, and the risk–benefit ratio must be favorable. There must be independent review of the study and subjects must receive informed consent. Finally, subjects must be treated with respect, including confidentiality, monitored progress, and the ability to withdraw. Additional ethical issues arise about treatments. Should comparison groups receive placebos or conventional treatment? Under what conditions can high-risk treatments be used? Ethical standards also arise in the analysis of results. In addition to "data-dredging", ignoring issues such as statistical power and experiment-wise alpha when planning a study is unethical. Similarly, the use of sample sizes that are smaller or larger than necessary puts subjects at inappropriate risk because the study either has insufficient subjects to find a difference or it has more subjects than were needed to find that difference. Finally, unethical communication practices are possible. The presentation of results in graphs can be misleading. In addition, inappropriate authorship and multiple publication of results are unethical practices. It is the discipline that must set the standards for research.

As physicians, we are also faced with ethical concerns related to our dual roles as physician and investigator. When we interact with patients who serve as both patients and research subjects, our boundaries and responsibilities become clouded. These sometimes-conflicting roles must be recognized and dealt with (Slatkoff *et al*, 1994). Only the discipline can set such standards (*see* Box 2.1).

Box 2.1 Ethical Issues in Conducting Primary Care Research

Study Conduct
- Possible study benefit
- Scientific validity
- Sampling procedure
- Risk–benefit ratio
- Independent review
- Informed consent
- Respect for subjects
- Treatments and controls

Statistical Issues
- Data dredging
- Ignoring type I and II errors
- Use of inappropriate sample sizes

Communication
- Misleading graphics
- Inappropriate authorship
- Multiple publication of results

Environment

The research environment includes many aspects that encourage research. Because these aspects fall under the purview of the department or residency, they are the responsibility of the research director and will be the subject of most of this book. Thus, "research environment" includes the research setting, research tools and resources, a milieu that includes stimulation by colleagues as well as collaboration and consultation, and opportunities for communication (Geyman, 1978).

Attitudes

Although the discipline and departments can endeavor to foster a passion for inquiry in family physicians via such resources as the Family Practice Inquiries Network (Dickinson *et al*, 2000), personal attitude ultimately rests with the individual. Curiosity, skepticism, and honesty are necessary for conducting quality research. However, awareness of the limited state of knowledge and an interest in learning from every patient must also be present. Physician-researchers must also appreciate the role that they play in research, must value their own observations, and must accept a personal responsibility for advancing the discipline (Geyman, 1978). In reality, there is little difference in the processes applied by clinician and investigator. Flexner (1910) said:

> the investigator . . . observes, experiments, and judges; so do the
> physician and surgeon who practice their art in the modern spirit. At

bottom, the intellectual attitude and process of the two are or should be identical. Neither investigator nor practitioner should be blinded by prejudice or jump at conclusions; both should serve, reflect, conclude, try, and, watching results, continuously reapply the same method until the problem in hand has been solved or abandoned.

Hence, the attitudes needed by the investigator are those that should already be present in the physician.

This recognition that the individual, the department/residency, and the discipline are responsible for different aspects of the research climate speaks to the model for research productivity espoused by Bland *et al* (2005). They suggest that productivity is dependent upon three pillars – the individual, the organization, and leadership. However, recognizing the local stresses and limitations placed on departments and residencies, the discipline could focus its energy beyond that of setting standards, working to promote productive non-local environments (e.g. national conferences, networks) and shaping appropriate attitudes through socialization.

Synthesis

In this chapter, we have noted that the climate for primary care research at academic health centers is not supportive. The climate for research is also less than optimal within the discipline. Unfortunately, the standards to be set and the attitudes needed for research are beyond the control of the research director. Although he/she can set local standards and work to foster attitudes favoring research, these may realistically rest with others. It is the local environment over which the research director appears to have some control. Yet, authority over the departmental milieu often rests with the chair or even the dean. All you can do, as research director, is to provide as supportive an environment as is possible while striving to foster the highest methodological and ethical standards within your faculty, realizing that your ability to achieve this will be limited. We are then ultimately left with the question of what is the role of the research director, with limited authority, in providing a nurturing environment for research within an academic health center and discipline that are less nurturing?

## Chapter 3

Whose Job is it? The Role of the Research "Director"

Vignette

Fresh from her clinical rotations, A.Z. was in a quandary, pressured to begin the hunt for a residency program but uncertain about what discipline to choose. She had entered medical school certain that she wanted to enter family medicine, happy to spend her career forming close relationships with her patients and caring for families. But now, she wasn't so sure. During every clerkship, at least one faculty member had told her that "she was too smart" to go into family medicine. Residents denigrated "local medical doctors" and the medical school still limited the hospital privileges of the family medicine faculty. And the fact that the Department of Family Medicine was still searching for a chair was very concerning. Did she really want to subject herself to such an environment?

An active, vibrant research program is not an accident, but rather a concerted effort of many people. However, different people play different parts in constructing this environment. The dean controls the environment within the academic health center, as the chair controls that of the department. Even the individual investigator is part of the environmental menagerie. So what role does each play and what is the role of the research director?

Role of the Dean

As discussed in Chapter 1, the academic health center does not always serve a nurturing role for clinical researchers, especially those in primary care. The pressures on the academic health center are great, and specialists often denigrate primary care research.

Although the dean's leadership style may be unrelated to scholarship (Wakefield-Fisher, 1987), the dean is responsible for encouraging research development among primary care departments, and for controlling the distribution of resources (Bawden, 1983). Through example and intolerance of behavior that destroys mutual respect, the dean can address denigration of primary care research by specialists. In addition, the dean can actively promote multidisciplinary research, and reward collaboration between primary care and specialty researchers.

The dean must also ensure that resources are provided that not only promote clinical research in general, but ensure that primary care research is supported. Thus, a strong grants management office can facilitate grant submission for all clinical researchers, but a grants management office that is facile with Agency for Healthcare Research and Quality (AHRQ), and Health Resources and Services Administration (HRSA) grants is especially helpful to primary care researchers. In addition, the Institutional Review Board (IRB) must understand the issues relevant to primary care research and, preferably, include primary care researchers on its board. Finally, the promotions and tenure policies at some institutions set standards, which are attainable only by basic scientists and an occasional specialist. Thus, the dean must ensure that promotion and tenure standards recognize the reality, demands, and opportunities of academic primary care, providing comparable rewards to productive researchers of every discipline. The promotion and tenure committee should include primary care faculty on its membership.

Direct financial support from the dean can also facilitate primary care research. Most deans have discretionary funds that could support research development in primary care departments. Also, policies concerning the distribution of indirect funds from grants could support primary care research.

Role of the Chair

The chair may represent the most important individual in the development of research within a department. Support for research should ultimately depend upon support from the chair. In the early stages of development, the chair may need to look to other departments within the institution to assist in fostering support and recruitment (Bland *et al*, 1993).

A productive organization depends upon the characteristics of the individual researchers, features of the departmental environment, and leadership. Whereas the characteristics of the individual researchers are the responsibility of the researchers themselves, and the research environment is the responsibility of the research director, leadership is usually the responsibility of the chair. To create a supportive environment, the chair needs to establish a research orientation within the department. He/she should establish clear research goals, and a decentralized structure and networks that support research. In addition, the chair needs to use a participative leadership style that encourages others to share information and ownership, while working together toward departmental goals. These supportive activities help to create a pro-research culture within the department.

In addition, the chair is instrumental in the recruitment of a research director and a core of productive research faculty (Bawden, 1983). Recruitment or development of a core of productive researchers is essential for success. If the chair has a scholarly reputation, it will enable him/her to influence others in the development of a pro-research culture and in the recruitment of productive researchers. If the chair does not have a scholarly reputation, then it is essential that the research director does.

The chair is also particularly important to faculty early in their career development. The chair is responsible for overseeing each faculty member's career development. He/she must not only ensure a collegial departmental environment with a research orientation, but should encourage collaboration and carefully assign the faculty member to committees. The chair should communicate expectations for performance via setting goals coupled with an annual review of progress. He/she must ensure that each faculty understands the promotion process, and should consider flexible timelines for faculty on tenure tracks, even seeking to stop the "tenure clock" if necessary. Thirdly, the chair should support the faculty member's scholarship through networking and provision of resources such as travel funds, pilot study support, personnel, and acquisition of institutional resources. Finally, the chair should encourage balance in the life of the faculty member: balance between professional and personal life.

Role of the Investigator

Despite support from the dean and department chair, a faculty may not participate in scholarly activities. Obviously, faculty must take the support provided to them and use it to pursue scholarship. Productive departments often have written or unwritten expectations that all faculty be involved in scholarly activities. Faculty must internalize such expectations so that scholarship is expected of themselves by themselves. Not only do such policies promote a culture of scholarship and a collegial environment, but such a culture may spill over into residency training as well. In addition to expectations of research and commitment of the faculty, they must dedicate themselves to the attitudes and standards discussed in the previous chapter.

Role of the Research Director

The role of the research director is both local and communal. He/she is responsible for the development of the individual faculty scholars as well as the community of scholars within the department. At times, these dual responsibilities conflict, requiring a balancing act based upon priorities and input from the chair.

Because the production of high-quality research depends upon the internal commitment of the researcher, the research director is not a "director" at all, but rather a co-ordinator and facilitator. Early on in the development of the discipline, the chair assumed the responsibility for providing a supportive environment and development of researchers. However, as medicine has become more complex and challenging, chairs have had less time to commit to these activities. Thus, it frequently falls to the research director to meet these responsibilities of the chair as well as those of the research director.

Even with the support of a scholarly chair who is dedicated to providing support for research and recruitment, the facilitative role of the research director is challenging. As a leader, the research director must set standards, encourage diversity, identify options, and provide support (Baldwin, 1983).

Policy setting and role modeling accomplish the setting of high standards (quality, productivity, ethics) for the department. Departmental policies can set expectations for individual productivity, and require review of protocols to ensure quality and ethical treatment. However, role modeling these standards may be even more effective than policy setting. Although the measure of effectiveness of a research director rests with *departmental* rather than *personal* productivity, the research director must be seen as a productive scientist, to establish his/her credibility and set standards for others.

Although there is a rationale for establishing a narrow departmental research agenda, encouraging diversity is important to the vitality of the departmental research endeavor and the discipline as well. This is especially true early in the department's research development. The concept of academic freedom is no less important to academic primary care than it is to the rest of scholarship. Academic freedom in departmental research means encouraging all research, not just that which has obvious clinical relevance. It also means displaying respect for everyone's ideas and resultant scholarship. Finally, academic freedom means a commitment to the provision of constructive critique of each other's work (Holloway and Bland, 1984).

The research director must assist faculty in identifying options to the challenges faced in the planning and conduct of research. No research study is perfect; all studies represent a balance between internal and external validity, between the ideal investigation and the reality of limited resources. The research director must be able to arbitrate this balancing act and assist investigators in identifying ways of maximizing their research pursuits.

Finally, the research director is key in securing and providing administrative support for research projects and the career development of investigators. Preferably, the research director should have access to personnel (e.g. research assistants) and financial resources that can be made available to investigators to support pilot studies and encourage travel to national meetings. However, the supportive role of the research director does not end there. The research director has direct responsibility for the day-to-day research environment. Thus, the research director is responsible for ensuring that faculty receive review, evaluation, and feedback on their research and career progress. It is also his/her responsibility that the environment provides opportunities for expanding the abilities of researchers through faculty development, collaboration, and mentorship.

Synthesis

Thus, for a department and individual faculty to be truly productive, the dean, chair, faculty, and research director must meet their obligations. Obviously, without faculty commitment, *no* research is possible. The research director can try to facilitate research without support from the chair, but a highly productive department is unlikely without the chair's support. In fact, establishing a new research emphasis within an established department without the *active* support of the chair is nearly impossible. Similarly, without support of the dean, the ability of the chair to promote departmental research is limited.

But the research director develops and implements the research development plan, translating the chair's research vision into research reality. He/she must provide leadership in terms of standards and encouragement at both departmental and individual levels. He/she must serve as a role model of productive scholarship. Finally, he/she must provide the resources for research.

It is the research director's job to nurture research at the individual level, allowing it to percolate up to the levels of the research team and the department, while focusing individual efforts to maximize the group output. This multiplicity of inter-level encouragement and steerage can only be orchestrated with a firm but non-authoritative hand.

## Chapter 4

Meeting the Administrative Responsibilities of the Research Director

Vignette

The research environment "sucked"! When C.V. had joined the department as research director, he had no idea how isolated the departmental researchers were. Although being individually very productive and respected, these investigators collaborated only with faculty from other departments. Attendance at departmental functions designed to share ideas and provide positive critique of manuscripts was poor at best. There wasn't even email traffic, announcing new funding opportunities or calls-for-papers. If someone landed an R01 grant, there was no celebration. Who was responsible for this non-collaborative, isolationist environment?

Certain themes emerge from studies of "successful" departments of family medicine. First, they have a reputation for clinical excellence. Without this reputation, academic departments become isolated within their institutions due to lack of respect. In fact, without a reputation for clinical excellence, it is difficult to pursue the other themes. Second, successful departments are part of a school-wide curriculum, giving them a sense of unity with a greater structure. Successful departments also develop networks of support. Although this usually involves relationships within the institution, networks outside the institution are also important. The fourth theme is that of a scholarly presence within the institution. In academic arenas, departments are ultimately judged "academic" based on their scholarship. Scholarship within an institution often depends upon the ability to collaborate with members of other departments, thus depending upon the institutional networks of support. Finally, successful departments have a record of recruiting and mentoring the best faculty. Without a scholarly reputation, it is difficult for an academic department to recruit the best faculty (Taylor *et al*, 1991).

Although these themes are best developed within the host institution, there may be circumstances that prevent it. For example, the all-powerful chair of internal medicine may make it his life's work to squelch primary care, thus preventing the department's pursuit of these themes locally. It is possible to develop unity with a greater structure, networks of support, and scholarship outside the institution, within the discipline of primary care. But it is more difficult.

Although applied to *departments* of family medicine, these themes may also be relevant to the task of developing a "successful" division of research within a department or division of primary care. First, the division must have the reputation of producing high-quality scholarship – both research and non-research scholarship. Second, the division must not be isolated from the rest of the department, but rather part of the primary care curriculum. Third, networks of support between productive members of the division and those outside of the division must be established. Fourth, recruitment and mentoring of the best researchers is critical. Finally, a strong scholarly presence within the department is vital if the division is to be accepted and receive its share of the departmental budget.

To meet the administrative responsibilities of the position, the research director must focus on leadership, resource development, administrative structure, faculty development, and relationships (*see* Box 4.1).

Box 4.1 Responsibilities of the Research Director

Leadership
- Vision
- "Cheerleading"

Resource Development
- Organizational resources
- Functional development resources
- Personal resources

Administrative Structure
- Prioritization
- Committee structure
- Research committee
- Promotion and tenure committee

Faculty Development
- Skill development
- Recruitment
- Socialization

Relationships
- Chair
- Departmental faculty

Responsibilities of the Director

Leadership

The cornerstone of leadership is vision. Although it is possible for the chair to provide the necessary leadership for the research program, this is unlikely when the chair lacks research experience and is not fully committed to the generation of new knowledge. Hence, the research director must be able to provide direction to the research effort, identify priorities, and develop strategies to secure the vision.

Perhaps just as important, the research director must be prepared to assume the role of "cheerleader". The research director must consistently reinforce the research climate, reminding others of its contribution to the department and the discipline, rewarding scholarly pursuit, and constantly re-inventing the scholars within.

At a higher level, the research director must be involved in the development and support of primary care research within the discipline. Such active involvement will promote discipline-wide change in research attitudes while fostering exchange of ideas that will enhance the local process of research development.

Resource Development

Although proposed for development of academic departments, the approach proposed by Bland and Ridky (1993) can be applied to the initial development of divisions of research within academic departments. This approach focuses on the structures, processes, and attitudes that facilitate development of organizational, functional, and personal resources.

Organizational Resources

Assuming the organization has higher aspirations, the focus here is on cultural intervention, changing the way the department views itself. Changing a culture is a daunting task and requires structural changes such as sociotechnical and personnel policy change. However, making these changes usually requires consultations and team building (Bland and Ridky, 1993). The research director must have support of the chair to carry out these changes.

Functional Development Resources

Assuming that arming faculty and staff with the necessary skills will produce functional development, the focus here is on motivation and transition programs, changing the way the department operates. Improving efficiency and motivation requires structural changes such as job planning and incentive programs. Making these changes usually requires training and managerial skill development (Bland and Ridky, 1993).

Personal Resources

Assuming that the faculty has the basic characteristics required of investigators, the focus here is on counseling and individual development, changing the way the individual faculty member operates. Changing individual performance requires employee support from both the organization and the individual. Making these changes usually involves mentorship and workshops on self-management, creativity, and research skill development (Bland and Ridky, 1993).

Administrative Structure

Everything cannot be done at once; the research director must prioritize activities. The first priority is the development of a research culture within the department. We will focus more upon the development of departmental culture in later chapters. Second, the recruitment and development of faculty is crucial to the establishment of a core of productive researchers. Finally, once the research "engine" is in motion, the priority is to take the research effort to a higher level of productivity or excellence.

To facilitate the administrative development of research support, a committee structure may be important to:

1. demonstrate that the development of research is not the responsibility of only one person, the research director, but rather everyone's responsibility
2. provide for a diversity of innovative ideas and keep the research director grounded in what is possible in this environment
3. permit more energy investment into development than can be provided by one person.

A Research Committee can address these objectives and should include a diverse membership. Although initially the committee may focus on review of proposed research to ensure quality and patient protection, the committee should evolve into a cadre of investigators committed to development of departmental research, each committing energy to the achievement of research-related activities. Due to the broad interest in conducting research in primary care settings, investigators from outside of primary care may want to use primary care patients in research studies. This provides the research director with a means for involving external researchers in the development of departmental research. Such researchers can be asked to sit on the research committee, can be expected to have their research projects reviewed and approved by the research committee prior to implementation, and can be used to develop novice primary care researchers if such external projects require involvement of departmental faculty as a condition for access to primary care patients. A second committee that should eventually be formed is a departmental promotions and tenure committee. This committee will:

1. keep faculty appraised on developments in the promotion and tenure process
2. annually review the curriculum vitae of faculty to provide feedback concerning progress
3. shepherd faculty recommended for promotion/tenure through the application process.

Faculty Development

All faculty will need faculty development if a strong research effort is to be built. No matter how skilled and productive a faculty member may be, they will need support to maximize their productivity. All productive faculty need assistance with their instructional activities, and production and editing of manuscripts and grants. Special programs to address targeted needs are also necessary. All faculty need assistance with career planning (Bland and Ridky, 1993). It is the research director's responsibility to ensure that these faculty development opportunities are available.

In addition, the quickest means to the initiation of a productive research core is through recruitment. Once measurable essential qualifications for new faculty are identified and ranked, active recruitment begins. In addition to the qualifications identified and a track record of productivity, an essential characteristic in these initial core researchers must be that they are good collaborators and interested in mentoring. These are the researchers who will be critical to the development of junior faculty as collaborators and mentors.

New faculty, or newly developed researchers, must be socialized. This includes orientation to the department, the institution, and the academic side of the discipline. In addition, these faculty will need assistance and mentorship with their research and their writing (Bland and Ridky, 1993).

Relationships

Everything is dependent on relationship. The success of any research director depends upon relationships. The majority of department chairs do not rank research as a top priority or challenge of the discipline (Katerndahl, 1994), and the majority of department chairs do not have substantial research experience (Murata *et al*, 1992). Hence, the research director is faced with a dilemma. To change the departmental culture will require significant changes in the way the department functions. However, for functional changes to be made, the research director must have the strong support of the chair, the same chair who does not understand or highly value research. Hence, the relationship between the research director and the chair is critical to the success of the research director.

Second, the research director cannot build a productive research program alone. Departmental faculty must be interested in promoting scholarship, value what research may bring to their teaching and patient care, be willing to do things differently, and assist in the development of themselves and the rest of the departmental faculty. To do this, the research director must not only sell the faculty on the value of research to them and the discipline, but must show them that he/she holds to their core values of teaching and quality patient care. Only through this understanding will faculty be open to the research message.

Development of the Director

Because the position of research director requires expertise in research, teaching and mentoring others in research, and securing and administering resources, the director must have research, faculty development, and administrative skills in order to be successful (*see* Box 4.2). Although the chair can seek to hire an experienced director of research who already possesses these skills, more than likely the director will not possess all of these skills up front, but instead will need development. When developing research within a department not known for its scholarship, there may be an advantage to having an MD in the position to facilitate acceptance of the need and feasibility of research by other physicians. However, in departments in which research is already part of the culture, PhD directors may be advantageous because the lack of clinical responsibilities for PhDs enables them to commit more time to the directorship. This may be particularly helpful when trying to take the department's research to a higher level of productivity. Finally, because the research director should have an established record as a scholar, and experience in academic work, it is inadvisable to recruit recent fellowship graduates for the position; they lack the experience and maturity to meet the challenge, and their potential as scholars and leaders is being jeopardized.

Box 4.2 Necessary Skills for the Research Director

Scholarship
- Research skills
- Statistical skills
- Publication skills
- Grant-writing skills

Faculty Development
- Instructional skills
- Evaluation skills
- Mentorship skills

Administration
- Team-building skills
- Delegation skills
- Resource management skills
- Project management skills
- Negotiation skills

Skills Required

The most important qualification that the director must have is expertise and experience in research. The director should come to the position with research and statistical skills as well as a track record of publishing research. The research director must be viewed as a respected researcher if he/she is to lead other researchers.

Although it is important for the director to have either research fellowship or PhD training to ensure the research skills, grant-writing skills are also critical. This is important not only for the development of the director's expertise and credibility, but also for acquisition of infrastructure support grants. Most fellowships do not provide adequate training in grant writing, so this skill may have to be developed elsewhere.

Because a major role for the director is to educate and mentor faculty in their development as researchers, another skill that the director needs is that of faculty development. The director must be able to prepare and deliver instructional sessions, prepare handouts, and mentor novice researchers. Being able to assess needs and individualize instruction is particularly helpful for the director who must nurture the development of researchers at all levels of expertise and experience.

As director of a division within an academic department, the research director must be able to build teamwork, delegate responsibilities, allocate resources, and manage projects. These administrative skills are often ignored in directors, but may be the most critical to departmental productivity when resources are limited. These are not skills that are likely to be developed in fellowship training.

Finally, negotiation skills are critical. As mentioned above, most chairs do not have research experience and do not share the research director's sense of necessity for research. Although valued, research will probably be held in less regard by the chair than teaching or clinical care. This means that there will inevitably come a time when the research director will have to negotiate for resources and commitment that the chair will be inclined to give elsewhere. Although having negotiation skills prior to accepting the position will probably prevent later problems, there will be an ongoing need for such skills as resources become tighter. Some basic rules that will facilitate any negotiation are to negotiate face-to-face, seek the best possible agreement for all concerned, look at short-term needs but long-term relationships, be prepared and knowledgeable about all of the issues, anticipate others' needs and strategies, and reach a consensus. Such negotiations must be held initially before accepting the director-ship, and periodically thereafter as the need arises.

Skill Development

Although it is ideal for the director to assume the position already in possession of these skills, in many departments and programs, that is unlikely to happen. Even if true, the director must continually refine these skills. Therefore, the director must have a plan for his/her own development.

Once the director has assessed his/her own development needs, the director should first look locally for skill development opportunities. The institutional review board, office of grants management, computing resources office, and office of instructional development may offer such opportunities. In addition, the institution's office of human resources may offer classes dealing with adminis-trative skills. If the institution cannot meet the development needs of the director, the community may be able to; if so, this will be a less expensive alternative to opportunities at national meetings. The business community may offer training in business and administration while universities may offer opportunities for specific coursework.

We will discuss, in later chapters, opportunities at a national level to develop research, statistics, and grant-writing skills. While meetings focusing on medical business management may be able to provide the necessary training in adminis-trative and negotiation skills, primary care meetings may also be able to provide instruction in other areas. For example, faculty development skills can probably be acquired at faculty development workshops or meetings of the Society of Teachers of Family Medicine (STFM). In addition, both state chapters and the national organization of the American Academy of Family Physicians sponsor leadership skill development meetings that may be valuable for research directors. However, opportunities specifically targeting the needs of the research director are limited. Without a national organization of research directors, this need must be addressed elsewhere. Although the North American Primary Care Research Group (NAPCRG) does offer workshops aimed at research directors, these offerings are limited. The Department of Family Practice at the University of Missouri offers a workshop for research directors, with feedback tailored to the individual director based upon his/her situation. However, because the director's chair must partici-pate in this workshop, this opportunity may not be available to every director.

Perhaps the most important advice for research directors is to recognize and plan for their own ongoing development. They must continue to refine their skills as researchers, and must develop their skills as administrators and leaders.

Synthesis

This section has emphasized the need for primary care research, while acknowledging its lack of institutional support. It is the department's (and ultimately the research director's) responsibility to provide a supportive environment for individual and departmental scholarship. To do so, the research director must have or acquire research, leadership, resource and faculty development, administrative, and relational skills. This means that, not only must the growth of faculty be supported, but so also must the growth of the research director. Perhaps the greatest error made by research directors is the failure to ensure their own research support and personal development; it is sacrificed for the good of others when resources are limited.

Section II

Developing Individual Researchers

## Chapter 5

Lighting and Fanning the Flame

> ## Vignette
>
> D.U. was frustrated . . . and in a quandary. The patient's hot flashes sounded like classic perimenopausal symptoms, but her follicle-stimulating hormone (FSH) and luteinizing hormone (LH) levels were normal. Although he searched MEDLINE, he couldn't find any studies on the ultimate diagnoses among primary care patients presenting with complaints of hot flashes. When C.V. "mistakenly" walked through the clinic, D.U. asked him if he knew of any such studies. C.V. said that he knew of none but that it sounded like it had the makings of a good study. With a stricken look on his face, D.U. reminded him that he had never done any research, to which C.V. quickly replied that the deadline for small institutional grants was approaching and that he was more than willing to help with both the research and the grant writing.

The research director is ultimately responsible for the scholarly productivity of both the individual researchers and the department as a whole. In addition, the director must balance short-term versus long-term outcomes. Thus, at both the individual and departmental levels, the director must weigh whether to emphasize immediate productivity or long-term capacity. Covey (1989) suggests that, in general, an emphasis on productivity *capacity* pays more dividends in the long run than does an emphasis on short-term productivity. Thus, the research director must constantly support the ongoing development of both researchers and the department in terms of their capacity to conduct high-quality scholarship and compete for funding.

Reasons for Investigation

Research is a calling, a way of life. Extraordinarily stimulating, the quest for something new is an exciting adventure, likely to minimize the chance of "burnout". As with Will Pickles, Edward Jenner, James MacKenzie, and Curtis Hames, we are part of a greater quest. Science and investigation are the most honorable of endeavors, and a natural part of medicine. Few clinicians providing the close one-on-one care to an ill patient would rather do anything else besides the all-encompassing, spiritually rewarding passion that is medicine. Yet, if we are willing to relinquish some of the personal aspects of providing such care, we can actually touch the lives of considerably more patients through the conduct and communication of scholarship (Katerndahl, 2003). Do we not have a moral obligation to advance the science of medicine, to critically evaluate the care we provide, to learn something from each patient and then communicate that knowledge to the rest of the profession? As physicians, we have a duty to question, to investigate, to increase our depth of understanding.

The research tradition itself is the ultimate manifestation of humanity's quest for knowledge. The student seeks to learn all that is known; the researcher seeks to learn that which is unknown. Research is a process of shedding light, of illumination. It may be true that research can never *prove* anything; no fact is known with certainty. The answer to any research study always leads to a new question; there is no end. Yet, it is still a process of getting answers to questions and, no matter how small the increments may be, progress is made.

The honorable nature of this quest in modern research is characterized by the tenets of the scientific method. This method requires honesty, objectivity, and a skeptical approach. It is a process of *a priori* establishment of a method of testing a hypothesis. Participation in such a rigorous critical endeavor is worthy enough, whether or not a publication results, whether or not one gets the answer desired; the quest is the highest form of scholarship.

From both a practical and aesthetic standpoint, there are a number of reasons to pursue research. In addition, the reasons vary depending upon perspective of the discipline, the department, or the individual (*see* Box 5.1).

Box 5.1 Reasons for Investigation

Discipline
- Expands knowledge base
- Attracts state/federal support
- Fosters growth of discipline
- Defines specialty
- Achieves parity with other disciplines
- Prevents regression of practice

Department
- Source of funding
- Recognition by other departments

Individual
- Improves critical appraisal skills
- Improves clinical skills
- Needed for promotion and tenure
- Development of the academic self

From the standpoint of the discipline, research expands our knowledge and also attracts the recognition that comes with state and federal support. In addition, research fosters growth of the discipline and helps to define the specialty. Through research, the primary care specialties seek to achieve parity with the other specialties. These are the practical reasons for a specialty supporting research. From a more theoretical perspective, there is no question that, without research, medicine would tend to regress over time, losing its academic air and its viability.

At the departmental level, there are basically two reasons for encouraging research, both of a practical nature. Research activities represent one source of funding for any department. Realistically, research is rarely a source of significant revenue, and is providing a diminishing financial return. Perhaps more importantly, acceptance by other departments within academic centers is governed chiefly by their recognition of research productivity. Without research, a department will not be viewed within the medical school community as contributing to academic medicine, and consequently will not be fully accepted by the other departments. Patient care and educational service do not carry the same weight in academia as contributions in research.

No matter how much a specialty or department wishes to foster research, without individual reasons, research would not take place. The researcher must have a strong drive in order to justify the investment of time and energy into any research project. Reasons to conduct research probably apply to every clinical researcher. First, conducting research improves the researcher's ability to evaluate the medical literature, thereby increasing his/her clinical knowledge, as well as improving their ability to teach. Second, through research the investigator can improve his/her patient care skills by improving their effectiveness, clinical judgment, and diagnostic skills. The final practical reason is particularly important to academic physicians. The reality of the promotion and tenure process rests heavily upon research productivity. Physicians who hope for promotion had better be involved in scholarship. On a more aesthetic plane, research contributes to the development of the academic self – the inquisitive, scholarly portion of every physician dedicated to the pursuit of knowledge. When the age of modern medicine began, there was no dichotomy between clinicians and researchers. All researchers were first clinicians. A return to these early physician–scientist days is being espoused by medical groups as a way of ensuring viability and continued progression of clinical research.

From the individual's viewpoint, there are several reasons to be involved in research. But whether these are sufficient to justify the investment of time and energy can only be answered on an individual basis. The researcher is part of an honored tradition, a marvelous commitment to knowledge and growth . . . but at a cost. The first step in the research process is the acknowledgment and acceptance of that cost.

Forms of Scholarship

Scholarship can take several forms, each relevant to primary care. In addition to the traditional form of *discovery* as represented by our classical view of a research study, a second form of scholarship is that of *integration*, such as a critical review of primary research. Integration is very important to primary care because it takes the scraps of knowledge produced by research and makes sense of them as an integrated whole, providing new insights. Primary care physicians need integration to learn from the bits of basic and clinical research that relate to primary care. *Application* is the translation of research into the practice setting, as in a demonstration project, integrating the results of primary research into day-to-day patient care activities. Although application is a current emphasis at the federal level, this form of scholarship has been lacking in the past. Finally, *teaching* is the communication of the results of the other forms of scholarship to others; innovative teaching programs represent scholarship as well (Beattie, 2000).

Primary care physicians value all four forms of scholarship. Not only is there a need to understand the small bits of primary research, but integration of research speaks to the whole-person emphasis of primary care. In addition, the controlled environment in which much of the research occurs means that not all research is directly applicable to practice, or to all practice settings. Thus, the translation of research into practice is critical. Finally, because primary care physicians are heavily involved in the training of future physicians, the scholarship of teaching is also valued. As a director of research, the emphasis is upon promoting discovery; however, the other forms of non-research scholarship are just as valid and should be supported as well. The department cannot have a class system of faculty based upon the form of scholarship pursued.

Levels of Commitment

There is a difference between commitment to (verbal support for) research and active involvement in research. Using psychiatry as an example, only 49% of full-time faculty psychiatrists report being committed to research; most of these are associate or assistant professors (Atkinson and El-Guebaly, 1996). If we define active research involvement by time spent in research, authorship, and external funding, only 16% of psychiatric faculty is actively involved in research. Comparing those who are actively involved with those who are merely committed to research, we find differences in their perceptions about training. Although no differences in mentorship were found, the active researchers valued training in data analysis, statistics, and laboratory experience more, while those who were committed valued training in patient care and clinical investigation more (El-Guebaly and Atkinson, 1996).

Although the numbers would probably be lower among primary care faculty, the patterns may be the same. Among family practice residents, although 85% state that research experience is desirable, only 48% are interested in doing research, with 8% actively involved. The difference between these residents was in the progressive access to resources (time and research personnel) among those residents who were actively involved (Temte *et al*, 1994). Although building commitment to research is not sufficient to ensure active involvement, it is a necessary first step.

Building Commitment to Research: Dentistry versus Evangelism

As a group, a faculty may recognize the need for research and for their department's research program; however, individual faculty members without prior research experience rarely recognize the need for their own involvement in the research endeavor. Aye, there's the rub! There are two basic approaches to building individual commitment to research among previously "uninitiated" faculty.

The "research dentistry" approach seeks to bully faculty into research by emphasizing the lack of advancement without it, anesthetizing faculty as much as possible by minimizing the level of their research involvement and workload, and imposing sanctions for those not complying. The department chair must be firmly behind this approach if it is to produce results. Although forcibly extracting participation may lead to research data and papers, it will not produce researchers. For that, there must be commitment to the aesthetic reasons for research, a burning desire to seek answers. Desire does not come with bullying.

The alternate approach, "research evangelism", seeks to bring the uninitiated into the research fold through personal means. The steps in evangelism include:

1. persistent involvement at home or work
2. becoming a friend
3. timely and personal sharing of your experience and their perceived need
4. service as a partner (Luis Palau Evangelistic Association, 1988).

Translated into the activities of the research director, this means that the message about the need for involvement in research and its do-ability is conveyed repeatedly in a variety of work and social settings, to both individuals and groups. Second, the message will only register if the director is viewed as a productive member of the team, holding values similar to the rest of the faculty. Hence, the director of research must be involved in all aspects of the department including teaching, committees, and clinical care if appropriate. The third step is then a matter of timing, the "researchable moment". Although the director can share personal experience of how he/she got involved in research and its subsequent rewards at any time, identifying the need for research and its feasibility are most effective if presented in the researchable moment, when the faculty member is faced with a clinical situation, for which there is no evidence-based answer. These moments must be actively sought by the research director and seized upon quickly before the glow of enquiry fades. This may mean being available frequently in the clinic to identify these moments, or often informally discussing recent clinical cases. Finally, once the faculty member has expressed the interest in pursuing a research question, the director must facilitate that study every step of the way as a personal research consultant. This may mean providing advice on the human subjects' review proposal, assisting in instrument development, securing a research assistant, or providing statistical analysis; whatever resources or support are needed, the director provides.

The Transtheoretical Model of Behavior Change (Prochaska and DiClemente, 1986) can help in moving faculty members along. At the precontemplative stage, pressure is not applied; you merely emphasize the positive aspects of involvement in research. Once the faculty member is contemplating starting a research project, you seek to identify the barriers that are preventing that involvement and deal with them. *It is essential that the initial research study be simple, do-able, and will contribute to the literature no matter what results are found.* Once the faculty member is preparing for involvement, you need to commit to your support, provide necessary resources, and establish a timeline and start date for the study. Once the study is underway, the director must make sure that it does not stall, even if it means personal involvement to keep it moving. Once completed, the faculty member's commitment to research should be maintained by ensuring the reward for the current project (by getting it presented at a national meeting and/or published), and identifying the next study to be pursued. Only after the faculty member has become a self-starter can the director's involvement be relaxed.

Synthesis

Fostering commitment and involvement in research by faculty members not previously committed to it can be daunting but highly rewarding. You must start with a recognition that not all faculty can or should be equally involved, and that high-impact scholarship may not involve research (non-research scholarship). Sharing the reasons for involvement in research is not enough; getting faculty involved in research requires personal involvement and recognition of research-able moments as they arise during the provision of clinical care. But faculty members will only be open to your message if they first view you as a colleague with similar values to theirs. Initial studies will require intensive support and commitment of resources, and they must lead to rewards.

## Chapter 6

Characteristics of the Productive Researcher

> *Vignette*
>
> He had paid his dues, collaborating with senior researchers, co-authoring papers and piloting his own preliminary studies. It was time for E.T. to develop his own research independence . . . and he had just the idea with which to do that, novel and innovative, but critical to primary care. He spent time plotting out a sequence of studies to fully explore the area and then focused his attention on the first study, summarizing the study design, identifying needed collaborators, and outlining the first manuscript. Then he turned to the needed co-investigators, arranging a group meeting and ensuring that there would be benefits for everyone involved, hopefully working toward a long-term collaboration.

Although many factors have been cited for the inadequacy of primary care research, two of the frequently proposed reasons reflect directly upon individual faculty characteristics. Poor faculty preparation, and heavy clinical and administrative responsibilities are felt to be important reasons for the inadequacy of primary care research (Huth, 1986).

Family medicine researchers themselves corroborate this, citing lack of time and support as the two factors that most discourage their productivity. On the other hand, while about half of the researchers indicated that infrastructure and the availability of mentors/collaborators were encouraging factors, over 20% indicated that their enjoyment in research and desire to advance the discipline were also encouraging factors (Hueston and Mainous, 1996).

What makes a researcher productive? Recognizing that "productive" reflects a combination of publications and funding as yet to be defined, the answer to this question is a mixture of personality, characteristics, habits, and professional networking.

Personality

True scholarship depends upon the character of the scholar. To ensure openness and honesty, the scholar must have integrity. Truth in research requires honesty. Perseverance is necessary if the scholar is to demonstrate sustained productivity. Without perseverance, rejection of grant proposals and manuscripts will end productivity. Finally, the true scholar risks expounding new (and perhaps radical) ideas; for this, he/she needs courage (Aday and Quill, 2000).

In addition, researchers need particular attributes for particular stages in the research process. For example, to conceive an innovative study, the investigator needs creativity, curiosity, clarity, and the ability for lateral thinking. In addition to the compulsiveness required of anyone conducting a study, the investigator must have curiosity and an ability for conceptualization if he/she is to design the study. Data collection and co-ordination require co-operation and organization respectively. Data analysis demands clarity of thinking in addition to mathematical ability. Finally, to disseminate the results and concepts, the researcher must have persistence as well as writing and presentation skills (Curtis, 1980).

Characteristics

As research director, you must be concerned with the productivity of the department as a whole; for this, you must foster a productive environment. However, the research director should also be concerned with the development of the individual researchers. The productivity of such researchers depends upon certain characteristics. In addition to such things as early research training and advisors, and departmental support (to be discussed later), Bland and Schmitz (1986) found nine individual characteristics in productive researchers.

Socialization

Productive researchers are socialized to academia and their discipline. They understand the issues and values of their organizations, and are involved in activities of these organizations. Productive family medicine researchers are usually active members in the Society of Teachers of Family Medicine (STFM) and/or the North American Primary Care Research Group (NAPCRG).

Mentors

Having mentor(s) is a characteristic of successful researchers. Mentors are instrumental to socialization, collaboration, and networking. Productive researchers typically have had a mentor from early on in their careers and have often had multiple mentors.

Work Habits

Productive researchers have a track record of productivity, which began early in their careers. Such work habits may include structured time for writing and subsequent publications, evidence of organization, and a disciplined approach to their research.

In addition, the choice of an initial project is key not only to the success of the project, but to the ongoing commitment of the investigator to a research career. Initial projects *must* be successful if the novice researcher is to receive enough encouragement to keep at it. Thus, the initial project should be of interest to the researcher and contribute to the literature no matter what is found. In addition, novice researchers need to be committed to doing it right rather than doing it fast. Finally, new researchers often underestimate what a project will entail (Goldman,

1991). As research director, you must keep the novice grounded in reality while encouraging their interest and progress.

Professional Communication

Sharing ideas and the results of research are characteristic of successful researchers. Such professional communication whether through formal presentations or informal networks enables investigators to obtain feedback on their ideas and keep them informed about others' work.

Local Peer Support

Although it is possible for researchers to produce in an environment in which they alone are involved in research, the most productive researchers typically have peer support at their institution. Supportive peers provide critical feedback and emotional support when necessary. Local peers are often the source of mentors and collaborators.

Simultaneous Projects

In addition to supportive peers, productive researchers are typically involved in multiple projects at multiple stages. This ensures an ongoing flow of completed projects. Ideally, a productive researcher has projects in the formative stage and the funding stage, projects in which data collection is underway and data analysis is being performed, manuscripts being written, being reviewed, and in press. Such high levels of productivity usually involve a mixture of large sophisticated studies, small pilot projects, and scholarly non-research projects.

Sufficient Work Time

Although the time available for research may vary from 10% to 80% in "successful" researchers, the ideal committed research time may be at least 40%. This represents sufficient time to maintain a high level of scholarly productivity, while still maintaining local commitment and orientation. Researchers with 90% of their time devoted to research will not be involved enough in departmental work to be viewed as a member of the "team", contributing to the department.

Orientation

Similarly, productive researchers are not oriented only to external issues and organizations. Yes, this external orientation is part of the successful researcher, but he/she also maintains an internal orientation. For example, in addition to serving on national panels, the productive researcher also serves on the local admissions committee. Thus, they are viewed within the department as contributing members of the department.

Autonomy and Commitment

This internal orientation is evidence of the commitment that successful research-ers feel to their local institution. Successful researchers are actively involved in the activities of their institution. However, they also desire and display a degree of autonomy, the capacity to work on their own, pursuing their own line of study. Such autonomy is critical for the highly productive, innovative work of the successful researcher. The exception to this rule is the new investigator who often languishes for lack of direction if too much autonomy is provided. Thus, new investigators need mentoring and guidance to provide them with direction and ensure their early productivity, so critical to long-term development.

Seven Habits of Highly Effective Researchers

Successful researchers across disciplines exhibit the academic characteristics mentioned above. However, productive researchers also demonstrate a particular approach to life that carries over into their academic activities. Stephen Covey (1989) has applied his "seven habits" to everyone from administrators to teen-agers. The success of his books suggests that there is a universal message within those seven habits that applies to everyone, including investigators. Although Covey says that individuals must concentrate first on becoming independent before they can focus on interdependence with others, investigators often develop the other way around. Researchers often begin their careers as colla-borators under an experienced investigator, and only later pursue their own projects. However, collaborators can actually slow productivity. Goldman (1991) feels that success in research is inversely proportional to the number of collaborators. My experience indicates that highly productive investigators find that collaborators slow them down but keep them honest, prevent them from making mistakes, and improve the quality of the outcome. Less-than-productive investigators find collaborators keep them moving forward and promote produc-tivity. In either case, faculty members committed to a career in research must understand the research endeavor, and have some experience in planning and conducting studies before they can be valuable collaborators. Although new investigators and clinicians can serve as collaborators, their value to the research project is limited by their inexperience. Therefore, we will focus on becoming an independent investigator first and then on becoming a valuable collaborator (*see* Box 6.1).

Box 6.1 Seven Habits of Highly Effective Researchers

Developing Independence
1. Be proactive
   - Planning and support
   - Do-able projects
2. Begin with the end in sight
   - Anticipated study outcomes
   - Program of study
   - Productivity versus productivity capacity

3. Put first things first
   - Anticipate problems
   - Organization

Developing Interdependence
4. Think win/win
   - Emphasize the relationship in collaborations
5. Seek first to understand
   - Anticipate barriers to collaboration
   - When problems arise, focus on understanding the position of others
6. Synergize

7. **Renewal**
   - Immersion in new knowledge or methods
   - Application of what you learn to patient care

Developing Independence

Be Proactive

Research cannot occur without a proactive researcher. Research requires planning and support. On the one hand, being proactive means seeking out individuals who can help you develop as a researcher and scholar, and seeking out experiences that will help in that development. On the other hand, being proactive in a research project means planning. The research must be do-able. Hence, the researcher must focus on research that interests him/her, accessible study populations, and topics in which he/she can intervene based upon the results of the study.

Begin With the End in Sight

A researcher must know what outcome he/she expects in a study. In fact, many advocate preparing "dummy" tables for data collected when planning a study. It is the outcome that dictates the data collected and how it is collected. Therefore, the researcher must have the end in sight.

But having the end in sight applies to a higher level. It applies to the program of study – a series of studies in an area designed to improve understanding of the outcome under investigation.

In fact, taken a step further, beginning with the end in sight also implies that we consider preparing for what we may anticipate will be the next program of study and to facilitate our research in general. Covey suggests that productivity consists of a balance between promoting productivity and promoting productivity capacity (P/PC). Thus, as we move through our current program of study, we should anticipate what may be our next program of study and begin laying the ground work – forming relationships, skills, development activities. In addition, we need to look for ways to ease our research workload and promote efficiency in research conduct, manuscript preparation, and grant writing.

Put First Things First

The concept of putting first things first relates to how the researcher spends his/ her time. The successful researcher plans far enough ahead to anticipate potential problems and avert crisis. If activities are classified by their importance and urgency, then the productive researcher avoids most activities in the urgent and non-urgent unimportant categories, focusing instead on important activities. However, the truly productive researcher spends little time on important urgent activities because he/she has concentrated their attention on important but non-urgent activities (Covey's quadrant II), thus minimizing the occurrence of urgent but important activities (crises). Researchers must be this organized and vigilant to prevent crisis management, a management strategy guaranteed to lead to incomplete or invalid studies, frustration, and unsuccessful research careers.

Developing Interdependence

At some point, an investigator's vision is going to exceed his/her skills, and collaboration will be essential if the program of study is to be addressed. Collaborators can broaden opportunities, provide skill sets, and share the work-load. Collaborators can contribute to problem definition, funding, instrument development, data collection or analysis, and interpretation (Irvine *et al*, 1990). In fact, faculty members who have been good collaborators in the past tend to be offered authorship on publications even with minimal involvement on the project (Mainous *et al*, 2002). However, by their very nature, collaborations pose challenges. Not only may egos and politics interfere, but collaborations require time and open communication if they are to succeed. Hence, you must be selective in choosing collaborators, focusing on their expertise and ability to work honestly with others.

Think Win/Win

Successful collaborations involve common goals, deadlines and flexibility, and early identification of roles. Within a supportive system, successful collaboration begins with researchers of character, which enables the development of trusting relationships and agreement. Everyone must benefit from the collaboration. Covey's "Win/Win or No Deal" approach is appropriate for collaborative relationships as well. Collaborators will only contribute if they perceive that they benefit fairly from the collaboration.

Seek First to Understand, then to be Understood

However, collaborations often go awry. Collaborators can be overly critical and get the task off track. They can become territorial or proceed on their own. Too often, collaborators just don't do their share of the work.

In addition to organizational barriers, which can decrease support for collaboration, other barriers exist. Professional barriers can include value systems, motivation, roles, workload, and history. Potential personal barriers include defensiveness, lack of creativity and initiative, unreliability or inflexibility, and poor communication (Irvine *et al*, 1990).

If problems arise within a collaborative relationship, the team must first listen to and acknowledge each collaborator's perception, and then diagnose the problem. Only then can a solution be sought.

Synergize

Synergy within collaborations cannot be programmed and does not develop overnight. It comes from a long relationship among collaborators of different backgrounds, and reflects a high level of trust and co-operation, which, in turn, leads to high levels of communication and new perspectives. In synergistic relationships, the group is more creative than its members are individually. In complexity science terms, synergy represents the emergence of new properties out of the self-organization inherent in a strong collaboration.

Renewal

Renewal can exist on more than one level. At one level, focusing upon pursuit of a program of study, renewal involves the periodic immersion in new knowledge or methods to further enhance the study.

However, on another level, renewal involves application of research findings. Research, teaching, and clinical care can reinforce each other. Potential burnout of the full-time researcher can be avoided by applying the knowledge learned through study to the patient care provided, and the teaching delivered to residents, students, and colleagues. In addition, such sharing of research results keeps investigators grounded in the reality of academic medicine and society.

Professional Networks

Professional networks consist of a number of colleagues committed to a professional objective. They serve a number of functions. In addition to providing general support and stimulation, networks serve a teaching function. They provide linkage within the institution and discipline, which fosters access and opportunities, information flow, and troubleshooting. Finally, networks promote research opportunities. Although research networks require energy, expense, and negotiation to maintain, and decrease individualization, networks have many advantages. Networks alleviate isolation, and promote new ideas and collective creativity. They allow access to larger study populations, to the most recent work, and to review panels. They allow for a greater skill set and can improve efficiency. Networks can create energy for projects and sustain motivation. Finally, research networks can promote better understanding, recognition of errors, and a means of critique.

Professional networks form through relationships among faculty within an institution, with former students, and within professional associations. They are usually maintained via communication through telephone, fax, and email as well as during professional conferences.

The effects of professional networks upon the individual faculty member can be dramatic. Not only can networks lead to more and better research, but they can ultimately promote productivity and satisfaction, which in turn can lead to income, awards, and promotion, and finally professional success (Hitchcock *et al*, 1995). Without professional networks, the academic scholar is a lone voice in the dark, compromised and unappreciated, at high risk for burnout. Academia is a social career; scholarship is based on peer review and support. "Lone rangers" are not likely to be successful.

Synthesis

Although the possession of a productive personality along with the development of characteristics, habits, and networks does not guarantee productivity, they are undoubtedly interrelated. Review of a diverse literature suggests that productive researchers share similar professional characteristics as well as habits that promote both independence and interdependence. Once these characteristics and habits are in place, professional networks serve to release the inherent productivity within the researcher.

The truly productive scholar is a master of multitasking and time management. Every scrap of time – in airports, awaiting meetings, between appointments – is utilized on some project. He/she is proactive in all things, spending a large proportion of time in Covey's quadrant II (important and non-urgent), always focused on future development. Thus, deadlines are not challenges, but are benchmarks, rungs on the ladder of scholarly progress. How does the research director go about developing such investigators?

## Chapter 7

Developing Research Skills in Individual Investigators

> ## Vignette
>
> She was new to the department, fresh out of fellowship, but F.S. already had plans to build a well-funded career over the next five years, with the support of her new chair. Based on the research productivity literature, she decided to limit her national presentations and internal collaboration, but rather to focus on building her publication track record and national service. Although tempted to eliminate her non-research scholarship and grand rounds presentations, she decided not to do that, but to use those activities to share her ideas with others and elicit their critique.

A primary role of the research director is the development of the investigators within the department. This not only includes the acquisition of basic research skills by the novice, but also the enhancement of research skills by the seasoned investigator.

The exact skills needed depend upon the researcher's role in the department. Thus, the researcher–teacher devotes equal time to teaching and research. He/she is capable of conducting moderately sized projects and serves as a role model to others. The researcher devotes most of his/her time to research with minimal teaching responsibility. He/she conducts major studies and is responsible for mentoring others. Finally, the research team member serves as a co-investigator and is mentored by others but has teaching as their primary responsibility (Watson, 1990). The skills needed to function in each role may be different (*see* Table 7.1). Both productive and less productive researchers rate the importance of research, writing, and research administrative skills similarly (El-Guebaly and Atkinson, 1996).

Table 7.1 Skills Needed Based upon Level of Research Experience

Novice	Intermediate	Experienced
Project Management Skills	Project Management Skills	Project Management Skills
Career Planning Skills	Career Planning Skills	Career Planning Skills
Research Skills	Research Skills	Research Skills
basic research skills	advanced research skills	R01 grant-writing skills
statistical skills	small grant-writing skills	innovative
presentation skills	theory development skills	methodological skills
writing skills		

What Skills are Needed?

Novice Researcher

Although all investigators need to have project management and career planning skills, novice researchers have a particular set of technical skills, which they need to master. These include basic research and statistical skills as well as presentation and writing skills. Investigators must be trained in these basic skills (Goldman, 1991). In a study of psychiatry researchers, those who were committed to research but less productive ranked the importance of training in clinical investigation and patient care as more important than did productive investigators (El-Guebaly and Atkinson, 1996).

Experienced Investigator

In addition to the basic technical skills of the novice researcher, the intermediate-level researcher needs to develop basic grant-writing skills and advanced research skills. Of particular importance, the intermediate-level researcher needs to also be able to use and build theory based upon research findings. At the experienced level, researchers need advanced grant-writing skills and to be able to use or develop innovative methods to address the complex research questions inherent in research at this level. Often, investigators must undergo a period of retraining mid-career (Goldman, 1991). Productive psychiatry researchers rated training in data analysis and laboratory experience as more important than did less productive investigators (El-Guebaly and Atkinson, 1996).

Strategies

Novice Researcher

Novice researchers need an extended, yet structured, period of instruction (Bland and Schmitz, 1986). Fellowship training is the primary method of providing this instruction (Mainous, 2003); the duration depends upon the research role the investigator seeks. Generally, a one-year fellowship is sufficient for those preparing for small projects or for collaboration on major projects. A two-year fellowship is usually recommended for faculty preparing to serve as principal investigators on major research studies and 2–3-year fellowships are recommended for those wanting to compete for R01 funding. Fellowship training is a consistent predictor of scholarly productivity.

Another strategy for development of research skills in novices is participation in research methods conferences. Attendance at the Primary Care Research Methods and Statistics Conference in San Antonio correlated with increased scholarly productivity (publications, presentations, and grants) compared with non-attendees. In fact, the more conferences that were attended the greater the productivity. Although these findings were also seen in intermediate-level researchers, the effect was greatest in novice investigators (Katerndahl, 2000a). However, for conference attendance to have its optimal effect, regular attendance at an ongoing conference is recommended.

Even local faculty development programs can be effective. In a survey of faculty development programs, junior faculty that participated in faculty development emphasizing academic project activities (working on academic projects, collaborating, receiving feedback and mentoring) reported significantly more professionally helpful relationships with mentors, peers, consultants, and colleagues. They also reported more professional socialization (career management, networking, and academic norms) due to the participation in these faculty development programs (Morzinski, 2005).

Experienced Investigator

Once an investigator has a track record of successful investigation, ongoing developmental needs may arise. Thus, seasoned investigators need to continue to grow methodologically. Networking and collaboration often leads to the awareness of previously unknown methodologies. Increased sophistication in the research questions asked leads to the need for increased sophistication in the methods employed. Such variety is essential for the growth and vitality of the seasoned investigator.

Not only does such growth develop as a result of collaboration and networking, but it can be fostered as well. Chairs can assign faculty varied professional activities and can vary their teaching responsibilities. Faculty can be given special projects or engage in brief periods with a specialized focus as a means of varying activities and duties. Finally, temporary non-academic assignments can also be used to stimulate varied interests and growth (Baldwin, 1983).

What to do about these newly developing needs for growth is another matter. Traditionally, sabbaticals served this purpose, but sabbaticals are not generally part of the academic medicine culture. However, brief focused fellowships are available and visiting professorships may also serve this purpose. The National Institutes of Health (NIH) offer K Awards for mid-career investigators for such a purpose, but these investigators must have previously been R01-funded. Exceptions are the K08 and K23 grants, mid-level career development awards for clinical and patient-oriented research. In addition, academic medicine is beginning to recognize this need. Concentrated programs such as the North American Primary Care Research Group's (NAPCRG's) Grant Generating Project offer the established researcher the opportunity to further their development. The Grant Generating Project seeks to take seasoned investigators without R01 success, and teach and mentor them through the process of acquiring their first R01. Its success is well documented; in four years, 58 grants were submitted for $19.3

Table 7.2 Multiple Regressions of 2-Year and 5-Year Outcomes (Ferrer and Katerndahl, 2002). Reprinted with permission from the Society of Teachers of Family Medicine, www.stfm.org

Predictor (Betas)	2-Year Outcomes			5-Year Outcomes		
	Grants	Presentations	Publications	Grants	Presentations	Publications
Baseline Activities						
Baseline Collaboration (no. of studies)						
external	−0.017	−0.003	−0.052	−0.052	−0.079[a]	−0.005
internal	−0.228[a]	0.002	−0.195[a]	−0.321[a]	0.096[a]	−0.171
Baseline Studies (no. of studies)						
research	0.313[a]	0.240[a]	0.347[a]	0.158	0.386[a]	0.502[a]
non-research	0.248[a]	0.309[a]	0.221[a]	0.257[a]	0.096[a]	0.073
new research	−0.021	−0.063	0.004	−0.030	−0.015	−0.116[a]
Baseline Outcomes (no.)						
presentations	−0.237[a]	−0.135[a]	0.240[a]	−0.151[a]		0.040
publications	0.139[a]	0.343[a]		0.494[a]	0.119[a]	
major publications	0.034			−0.295[a]	−0.213[a]	
grants submitted		0.060	0.017		−0.001	0.040[a]
grants as PI		0.071	0.005		−0.061[a]	0.074

Professional Status						
Assistant Professor (yes)	−0.074	−0.031	−0.017	−0.059	−0.139[a]	−0.050
Full-Time (yes)	0.017			0.094[a]		
Tenure Track (yes)	0.069	0.074	−0.042	0.081[a]	0.195	−0.019
Years Since Graduation (no.)	−0.264[a]	−0.206[a]	−0.212[a]	−0.226[a]	−0.216	−0.373[a]
Degrees (yes)						
non-MD degree	0.008			0.088[a]	0.201	
advanced degree		−0.050	0.273[a]		−0.242[a]	0.424[a]
Fellowship Training (yes)						
any fellowship or PHD					−0.217[a]	
1–2 years or PHD	0.234[a]	0.008	0.150[a]	0.263[a]		0.114[a]
Service Indices						
departmental	0.190[a]			−0.073		
national	−0.082	0.046	0.233[a]	0.132[a]	0.456[a]	0.244[a]
grand rounds (no.)	0.220[a]	0.283[a]	0.129[a]	0.235[a]	0.410[a]	0.146[a]
Demographics						
Male (yes)	0.201[a]			0.286[a]		
Marital Status (yes)						
divorced/separated	−0.026	−0.189[a]	−0.270	0.045	−0.361[a]	−0.335[a]
single						0.197[a]
Children at Home (no.)		−0.044	−0.010		0.064[a]	
Adjusted R^2	0.888	0.925	0.888	0.609	0.373	0.581

[a] $P \leq 0.05$.
PI: Principal investigator.

million and 19 out of 41 non-pending grants were funded (Campbell and Longo, 2002). Other projects using a similar design could be developed to meet other faculty needs.

Predicting Individual Productivity

Previous research on predictors of individual scholarship has focused on professional training (e.g. fellowships), research environment, and professional activities as predictors. The prevailing logic suggests that fellowship training, a supportive environment, and research activities are positive predictors, while administrative and patient care responsibilities are negative predictors. Does research support this and what are the implications?

Training

Compared with faculty without fellowship training, faculty with fellowship experience spend more time in research, are more likely to be published, and have more submitted and funded grants (Hueston, 1993b; Barnett et al, 1998; Taylor et al, 2001). Although self-reports from faculty who attended full-time and part-time fellowships were positive (Reid et al, 1997), faculty with at least one year of research fellowship training were more productive than those with less than one year of fellowship experience (Taylor et al, 2001). This supports the work of Ferrer and Katerndahl (2002), who found that fellowship training of at least one year or a PhD degree was associated with both two- and five-year scholarly productivity (see Table 7.2). Similarly, clinical pharmacy faculty involved in a 3-year scholarship program spent more time in research and collaboration than those who did not. In addition, their productivity was less influenced by chairs and resource support, and research experience (Jungnickel and Creswell, 1992).

Although a variety of fellowship programs exist in primary care, the two-year Robert Wood Johnson (RWJ) and National Research Service Award (NRSA) fellowships have received the most attention from researchers. However, these fellowship graduates were not very productive within the years following fellowship training. The NRSA graduates studied were involved in a median of three research projects (one as the principal investigator and one with funding) and had a median of zero publications (Curtis et al, 1992). Post-fellowship, both RWJ and NRSA graduates report low levels of research productivity. The explanation for this low level of productivity is the lack of resources and mentors, while being given administrative responsibilities (Perkoff, 1985; Curtis et al, 1992). Predictors of post-fellowship productivity among NRSA graduates included having a mentor, spending at least 40% of the fellowship time in research, and involvement in an NRSA fellowship in pediatrics or internal medicine; family medicine fellowship graduates fared poorer (Curtis et al, 2003).

Environment and Activities

The Faculty Activities and Research Environment Survey (FARES) found that scholarly success as measured by publications and funded research was associated with research activities and scholarly habits (Hekelman et al, 1995b). In an unpublished study within our department on the two- and five-year predictive validity of the FARES, local mentoring was related to the number of research and non-research scholarly projects. In fact, local mentoring was predictive of research presentations over the next two years, and grant submissions over the next two and five years. Current research activities were predictive of two-year research publications and five-year research presentations. Finally, scholarly habits were predictive of two-year research presentations and submitted grants (Katerndahl, 1995). In a recent study, Brocato and Mavis (2005) found that research environment was primarily related to grant submissions, but research time was associated with all measures of productivity. However, the most important correlate of publications and presentations during a two-year period was psychological and cognitive factors.

Although teaching and service are often said to inhibit scholarly activity, Ferrer and Katerndahl (2002) found that, in one department, patient care and teaching were negative predictors only of research presentations; they were positive predictors of publications and grants. This agrees with the reviews of Rhoades (2001) and Bland *et al* (2005). Similarly, although departmental service was a negative predictor of publications, it was a positive predictor of grants. In fact, the number of grand rounds presentations was a positive predictor of two- and five-year grants, presentations, and publications. National service to the discipline was a positive predictor for five-year scholarly outcomes. Megel *et al* (1988) also found that highly productive faculty spent significant time in administration and institutional service, but less time in teaching. Mularski and Bradigan (1991) found that directors and associate directors had high rates of publication.

Both research and non-research scholarly projects were predictive of two- and five-year presentations, publications, and grants (Ferrer and Katerndahl, 2002). When the research activity is dissected, as expected, the number of completed studies is predictive of all outcomes. In addition, the number of different stages (from planning to completion) represented by these studies was also predictive of most outcomes. However, the proportion of studies in data collection was inversely related to two-year publications, and both two- and five-year grants. The proportion of studies dropped prior to completion was inversely related to two- and five-year presentations (*see* Table 7.3).

Research presentations at national meetings are often subsequently published. Presentations at a nursing research conference are re-presented 34% of the time and published 13% of the time (Clickner *et al*, 1998). Presentations at STFM and NAPCRG fare even better; 48% are published within 4–5 years, with 56% published in family medicine journals (Elder and Blake, 1994). Highly productive faculty have many co-authored national presentations (Megel *et al*, 1988). Ferrer and Katerndahl (2002) confirmed that current research presentations were predictive of two-year research publications. In addition, although current publications were a negative predictor of two-year presentations, they were positive predictors of two- and five-year grants. These findings may support Bartle *et al* (2000) who found that current publications and presentations correlated, but writing and authorship status were negative correlates of presentations. High productivity among nursing faculty is predicted by research team involvement, preference for research over teaching, and for writing manuscripts and grants, co-authored presentations, prior research experience, and institutional service (Megel *et al*, 1988).

Table 7.3 Research Activity Predictive of 2- and 5-Year Productivity

Research Publications		Research Presentations		Grant Submissions As PI	
2-Year	*5-Year*	*2-Year*	*5-Year*	*2-Year*	*5-Year*
# Completed	# Completed	# Completed	# Completed	# Completed	# Completed
# Stages	# Stages	# Stages	# Stages	# Stages	# Stages
# As PI	# Planning	# Collection	(# New)	# Funding	(% Planning)
(% Collection)		% Completed	(% New)	(# Dropped)	(% Collection)
		(# Funding)	(% Dropped)	(% Collection)	
		(% Dropped)			

# As PI	Number of studies as principal investigator.
# Planning	Number of studies in planning stage.
# Funding	Number of studies seeking funding.
# Collection	Number of studies in data collection.
# Completed	Number of studies completed but active.
# New	Number of new studies.
# Dropped	Number of studies dropped.
# Stages	Number of stages (from planning to completion) represented by active studies.
% Planning	Proportion of studies in planning stage.
% Collection	Proportion of studies in data collection.
% Completed	Proportion of active studies completed.
% New	Proportion of studies that are new.
% Dropped	Proportion of studies that were dropped.
( )	Inversely related to productivity.

Synthesis

This work suggests that fellowship training, particularly that which includes an extended period of research, is associated with post-fellowship research productivity but is often limited by lack of mentoring and resources. Contrary to expectations, patient care, teaching, and administrative responsibility were often not detrimental to scholarship and, in fact, may serve as the focus for scholarship. National service was linked to five-year outcomes.

Local mentoring and scholarly habits were also associated with scholarly outcomes. As expected, these outcomes were strongly linked to current research activity, particularly to the number of different stages represented by current research. However, the proportion of studies in data collection or dropped had a negative impact on grants and presentations respectively. In addition, the outcomes were interrelated; presentations often led to publications, and publications often led to grants. Thus, the activities upon which a researcher focuses may differentially affect different outcomes. Time investment should be guided by long-term scholarly goals.

As research director, these observations suggest certain approaches to take when developing researchers. First, all activities – patient care, teaching, administration – are interrelated and can be used to focus and promote scholarship. All forms of scholarship – presentations, publications, grants – are interrelated and can be used to promote each other. Thus, optimal research involvement may *not* be 90% research time, leaving the faculty member with little non-research activity and contacts, isolating him/her from the rest of the faculty. Second, different factors affect different outcomes on different timescales. Thus, career planning is essential to determine how to focus activity to maximize a researcher's chance of meeting his/her goals on schedule.

## Chapter 8

Individual Resources: Mentors and Money

> ## Vignette
>
> G.R. joined the faculty after her fellowship and had already published three research papers in the past two years (and was feeling pretty good about her research career). Her mentor wasn't quite so pleased. H.Q. pointed out that, to develop a strong National Institutes of Health (NIH)-funded career, she needed early career development support. She currently had 20% of her faculty time for research. H.Q. suggested that her next project should focus on a K Award application.

Being Mentored

Successful researchers have a history of being mentored by researchers during their development. Having an influential mentor is a positive predictor of more than one publication per year (odds ratio, OR = 4.0) and serving as the principal investigator on a funded grant (OR = 3.1) among faculty who completed a National Research Service Award (NRSA) fellowship (Curtis *et al*, 2003). Academic faculty who have had a mentor rate their research skills, teaching and administrative support, and career satisfaction higher, and report more time available for research (Palepu *et al*, 1998). In fact, ongoing junior–senior researcher relationships are important for the continuing development of the investigator (Mainous, 2003). Although the role of the mentor will be addressed more fully in Section III, a mentor provides career guidance and opportunities, and serves as a sounding board on professional issues, facilitates networking, and encourages appropriate lifestyle management. Yet, only 54% of junior medical school faculty report having a recent mentor; only 61% report ever having a mentor (Palepu *et al*, 1998).

Role of the Protégé

Before entering into a mentor–protégé relationship, protégés must be proactive about their careers, identifying what aspect of their career needs development and what kind of assistance they need (i.e. teaching, socialization, nurturing, advocacy, or role modeling). Protégés need to have a focused content area and have identified experts in that field. Finally, protégés must be willing to engage mentors, sometimes more than one (Rogers *et al*, 1990; Stange and Hekelman, 1990).

When choosing a research mentor, protégés need to look for certain characteristics in their mentors. Mentors should be currently involved in funded research, and have a track record as well. Protégés should actually check the publication records of prospective mentors. Mentors must be able to provide quality supervision. Perhaps the best predictor of a successful mentoring relationship is the prior success of a mentor's relationships. Are the mentor's prior protégés currently in good academic positions and satisfied with their careers? Have these prior protégés secured funding, completed their research projects, and published their results (Goldman, 1991)? Matching mentor–protégé gender and race/ethnicity may also be important.

Once a mentor–protégé relationship has been negotiated, the protégé needs to actively participate in the experience. The protégé must know his/her goals and meet regularly with the mentor, listening to the advice given. Because the mentor must be critical of the protégé's work if the protégé is to improve, the protégé must avoid being overly sensitive. The relationship must be kept strictly professional, and any confidences shared by the mentor must not be betrayed. The mentor–protégé relationship will only work if the protégé is committed to the process.

Course of the Mentor–Protégé Relationship

The mentor–protégé relationship can last up to six years. After a 6–12-month initiation phase, the relationship enters a 2–5-year mentor–protégé phase. Once the formal relationship ''breaks-up'' after that, friendship often follows. The subsequent peer-oriented relationship involves the collegial sharing of information and may last a lifetime (Hitchcock *et al*, 1995).

The protégé can benefit tremendously from this relationship but must also be on guard for potential problems. Not only does a mentor–protégé relationship require time to develop, commitment to the process, and time to pursue, but the identification of the right mentor or mentors is not easy; inter-gender and inter-racial issues can pose problems. Once developed, the close dependency that results can go too far; the protégé must move from the early dependency into a mature independent trajectory. Protégés and mentors must watch for the development of overdependence. Similarly, although protégés must expect to ''pay their dues'' by contributing to mentors' projects, some mentors simply give bad advice and some may take advantage of protégés. Hence, protégés must watch for this and be willing to draw the line when they are no longer receiving commensurate benefits for the time invested. On the other hand, mentors may become disillusioned with protégés who repeatedly disappoint them.

Fortunately, such problems are the exception. The mentor–protégé relationship typically is an extremely valuable and productive one. As director, you must identify those novice researchers with potential for highly productive research careers, and assist them in forming mentor–protégé relationships. If appropriate mentors do not exist within the department (as is often the case in primary care), then mentors should be sought from other departments within the institution or even from other primary care departments outside the institution if necessary.

Funding Researcher Development

In 1992, more than half (51%) of all primary care research was unfunded. Federal and local agencies accounted for 17% and 7% of research, respectively. The discipline supported 12% of studies, and foundations and corporate sponsors each supported 7%. The figures for federal and discipline support are significantly different from those for other disciplines (Ruffin and Sheets, 1992). The funding support for family medicine research was even worse. Although NIH funding from 1984 to 1997 increased from $5.9 billion to $11.8 billion, the proportion of the NIH budget supporting family medicine research remained at 0.3–0.4%; support from the Agency for Healthcare Research and Quality (AHRQ) remained at about 4% of their budget (Campos-Outcalt and Senf, 1999). With funding support being so poor in primary care, we must seek to improve the funding situation.

In February 2005, a workshop was held, focusing on the development of sustainable NIH-funded research programs in primary care. The resulting recommendations included, first, having an external mentor and securing career development funding; second, developing a particular research method or theme and sticking to it – starting by defining a major idea and then attacking pieces of the problem. Third, time is critical. You need at least 50% research time and should avoid service on time-intensive committees (i.e. institutional review board). Use fellows and graduate students to supplement research assistant support. Fourth, attend national meetings attended by NIH representatives and seek their input. Fifth, focus on publications instead of conference presentations. Publications should have a common theme and each R01 grant should quickly lead to 5–10 publications with every research team member contributing. Finally, a sustainable program requires vision. Not only should R01s overlap, but carryover funds should be built in through rebudgeting.

Funding Research Projects

Unfunded research is supported by a variety of sources, including working extra hours (73%), other funded projects (63%), discretionary funds (56%), and clinical income (27%). The purpose of this unfunded research is usually pilot work (71%) or an extension of funded research (78%), but unfunded activity can also be necessary for supported projects (50%) or research in a new area (52%). Often, this unfunded research produces dividends. These projects typically lead to publication (80%) and/or funded research (54%).

Although typically we think of NIH funding when we consider research support, we must be open to other sources as well, especially for pilot projects. In addition to institutional and Veterans Administration grants, investigators should also consider pharmaceutical companies if projects can be tied to directions for new pharmaceuticals. Both small and large foundations can be sources of research funding; even the National Science Foundation will fund primary care research if the project is focused on basic understanding rather than treatment.

While being a junior faculty member (versus a senior faculty member) is a predictor of receiving institutional funding, faculty conducting unfunded research are typically principal investigators on funded research, spend over 35% of their time on research, and have institutional funding as well (Weissman *et al*, 1999). These numbers not only suggest that other clinical faculty also rely heavily on institutional and departmental support, but that the senior researchers may be better able to conduct unfunded studies, while junior researchers tend to rely on institutional support.

In addition to the predictors of research funding presented in previous chapters, it is important to realize that once the researcher has successfully competed for one NIH grant, future funding becomes easier. Of those investigators who received NIH funding in 1972 or 1982 and were followed for 10 years, only 40% received only one grant over the next 10 years. However, if an investigator received only one grant in a 10-year period, 93% of the time it was the only one they ever received; if at least two grants were received, 27% of the time no other grants were received (Rajan and Clive, 2000). The importance of developing a track record cannot be over-emphasized.

Thus, when seeking support for research, efforts must be geared to the researcher's level (Goldman, 1991). Novice researchers should seek support from their institution and agencies focused on supporting junior researchers. While senior faculty can concentrate on major funding, they also have the ability to conduct unfunded projects that can lead to major funding. To bring the novice researcher to the point at which they can compete for major funding, the novice must seek funding to further their research development.

Funding Researcher Development

HRSA funding, usually through the Academic Administrative Units' grant mechanism, can be used to support development of researchers. Wagner *et al* (1994) found that the level of such funding received by a department predicted the number of publications per faculty member, accounting for 16% of the variance. In fact, all four Health Resources and Services Administration (HRSA) training grant mechanisms can be used to support research via linking funding to the support of students or residents in research, to faculty development of research skills, or to development of a research environment within academic units.

Other mechanisms have specifically targeted researcher development. The Advanced Research Training program of the American Academy of Family Physicians (AAFP) and the Generalist Scholars' Program of the Robert Wood Johnson (RWJ) Foundation were successful programs designed for this purpose. Although both programs are coming to an end, their success may lead to future similar offerings. The primary funding mechanism for researcher development currently available is the K Award mechanism offered by the NIH and AHRQ. These awards focus on researcher development at all levels and have a higher funding rate than R01 grants. At this point in time, any primary care junior researcher considering a quest for NIH funding should seek K Award funding early in his/her research career.

In one study of 152 recipients of career development awards, 21 (14%) left the university; most were PhDs and half left within two years of the end of the award. This emphasizes the need for ongoing mentoring after the career development award expires. But the success of such awards cannot be denied. Over at least four years, 70% of recipients were successful in receiving continuous funding after the end of the award (Yip and Waxman, 1997). Such success speaks for itself.

Synthesis

Despite training and development, researchers must have certain resources in order to be productive. The most important resource for a beginning researcher is mentorship. Ultimately, however, the researcher (and the research director) must be able to fund research projects as well as researcher development. Grantsmanship should be taught early, and career development grants should be pursued soon after training. For a researcher to develop as an NIH-funded investigator, he/she should publish regularly and secure career development funding within five years of fellowship completion. It is the researcher's mentor (and ultimately the research director) who must ensure this happens.

But funding and research productivity are not the ultimate measures of the success of individual faculty members. Those measures are promotion and tenure.

## Chapter 9

Receiving Promotion, Getting Tenured

> ## Vignette
>
> I.P. was a team player, always filling in for any faculty member who was ill and unable to meet their clinic obligations. He had been teaching in the residency program for eight years, precepting residents, lecturing students, and providing care to his own patients. In fact, he would cover others' responsibilities while they attended national meetings. Now it was his time for some recognition because his chair had recommended him for promotion and tenure. Much to his chagrin, when the institution's promotion and tenure committee contacted his chair, they saw his contribution differently. Not only was he denied both promotion and tenure, but he was reminded that his tenure clock would expire in two years; if he wasn't awarded tenure by then, he would have to leave the institution!

Promotion and tenure (P&T) are the ultimate benchmarks of success, from the faculty member's standpoint. Department chairs look for fiscal solvency, growth, and reputation, but faculty look for recognition via promotion and institutional recognition via tenure.

At academic centers, promotion may depend upon factors other than scholarship and achievement. For example, among academic radiologists, men are more likely to be full professors, be on the tenure track, and to have grant support compared to women. Even when women are promoted to full professor, they have on average spent a year longer at the rank of associate professor (6.76 versus 5.64 years) (Vydareny *et al*, 2000). Similarly, compared with non-Hispanic whites, under-represented minority faculty are less likely to be promoted to associate professor (odds ratio (OR) = 0.68) and full professor (OR = 0.81) (Fang *et al*, 2000). Does this mean that the P&T process is governed by discrimination? Not necessarily; there may be reasons other than "discrimination" that result in fewer women and/or minorities in research rather than teaching and patient care training.

The fate of family medicine faculty improved from 1981 to 1989. During that period, promotion rates rose for all ranks, for MDs and PhDs alike, for faculty at all types of medical schools. The largest increases in promotion rates were for assistant-to-associate professor, for MDs, and for those at low-research public medical schools (Gjerde, 1994). These improvements reflect general changes in the P&T process in recent years.

The P&T process and criteria are in a state of change in academic medicine. In a 1998 survey of the 125 medical schools, only 11 did not offer tenure to clinical faculty. In fact, most schools (73%) offered non-tenure tracks. Those schools with tenure generally required achievement of tenure within seven years of appointment (59% of schools). According to Table 9.1, considerable change in tenure policies had occurred within the past three years (Jones and Gold, 1998).

Table 9.1 Changes in Tenure Policies (Adapted from Jones and Gold, 1998)

Change in Policy	Proportion of Medical Schools (%)
Modify faculty compensation	24
Lengthen pre-tenure probation	12
Modify promotion-tenure link	6
New faculty track	26
Periodic evaluation of tenured faculty	22
Periodic evaluation of all faculty	26
Redefine salary guarantee	11

However, there is also talk about eliminating tenure as an antiquated, irrelevant policy designed to ensure academic freedom, but unnecessary for clinical faculty. In addition, there is growing concern that, once received, tenure is abused, leading to decreased productivity. Hence, many academic centers have instituted post-tenure reviews to assess continuing productivity, and with the power to revoke tenure. Yet, studies of clinical faculty have demonstrated increased, not decreased, productivity after receipt of tenure. Although Waller *et al* (1999) reported that publications dropped after receiving tenure, Megel *et al* (1988) found that among nursing faculty members, post-tenure research publications rose from 2.4 to 3.5 per year, non-research articles rose from 3.3 to 3.9, and grants rose from 1.1 to 1.9. In fact, the relationship between increased research publications and receipt of tenure was most pronounced in the most active researchers. While currently inactive researchers had a drop in research publications before and after tenure (2.2 to 0.7 articles), those with low, moderate, and high productivity had rises of 1.6 to 3.5, 4.9 to 8.0, and 4.6 to 9.8 publications, respectively. Thus, there was no drop in productivity post-tenure, and the most productive faculty had the greatest increase in publications. Receipt of tenure apparently boosted their productivity.

Predictors of Promotion

Assessment of scholarship is based upon a sense of trustworthiness of the institution. Thus, the process must be open to scrutiny, the methods must be fair, the results must focus on growth, and critique must be ongoing and flexible (Aday and Quill, 2000). Various methods have been devised to measure scholarly productivity. Recently, the use of relative value scales to measure academic productivity has been proposed. Table 9.2 presents some of the relative values for scholarship on one such scale (Scheid *et al*, 2002). On this scale, a 1-hour consultation in an area of expertise counts 0.86 relative value units. By comparison, an invited national presentation counts 1.80 points, serving on a national study section earns 1.60 points, submitting an unfunded grant counts 13.31 points, and publishing an article in a national refereed journal as first

Table 9.2 Relative Values for Scholarship (Adapted from Scheid *et al*, 2002)

Product	Relative Value
Scholarly Activity	
Attending Research Presentation	0.4
Assisting Learner with Research for 1 h	0.68
Presentations	
national, refereed	1.71
national, invited	1.8
local, refereed	1.27
local, invited	1.12
CME presentation	1.14
public service presentation	0.89
Reviews	
critiquing colleague's paper	0.68
peer reviewer for grant/journal	1.01
peer reviewer for book	1.35
national study section	1.6
local study section	1.09
IRB meeting	1.13
mock study section	0.83
Consultation in Area of Expertise (1 h)	0.86
Administration	
program director	4.51
grant principal investigator	3.61
grant facilitator	2.49
editor for series of volumes	2.85
editor of journal	3.79
editor for series of papers	2.92
Grants	
Funded, Principal Investigator	30.23
Funded, Co-investigator	18.32
Approved, Principal Investigator	17.54
Approved, Co-investigator	11.21
Not Approved, Principal Investigator	13.31
Not Approved, Co-investigator	8.34
Publications	
Papers/Chapters	
refereed, national	
solo author	20.87
first author	16.62
co-author	11.8
refereed, local	
solo author	13.68
first author	12.0
co-author	8.22
non-refereed, national	
solo author	10.54
first author	9.8
co-author	7.3

Table 9.2 (*cont.*)

Product	Relative Value
Publications (*cont.*)	
non-refereed, local	
solo author	8.01
first author	7.27
co-author	4.61
unpublished report	
solo author	5.72
first author	5.31
co-author	3.34
Books	
solo author	28.25
editor	22.42
first author	21.91
co-author	19.4

CME: continuing medical education; IRB: institutional review board.

author counts 16.62 points. The problems with such productivity formulae include the interdependence of such measures, the lack of a qualitative perspective, and the failure to recognize the uniqueness of each faculty member's contribution (Grams and Christ, 1992).

Whether productivity formulae are used or not, promotion and tenure are based heavily on scholarly productivity in terms of publications, national presentations, and grants. For family medicine faculty, the trends are interesting. In 1981, successful candidates for promotion had more articles published compared to unsuccessful candidates (7.4 versus 3.4 at the associate professor level and 11.0 versus 5.0 at the full professor level). Although there were no differences in book chapters at the associate professor level, those promoted to full professor published more chapters than those not promoted (1.7 versus 0.5) (Gjerde *et al*, 1982). By 1989, successful MD candidates for promotion to associate professor differed little from unsuccessful candidates in the number of publications. However, at the full professor level, successful MD candidates had 17.2 publications versus 15.4 for unsuccessful candidates (Gjerde, 1994). Overall, the number of publications by successful candidates had increased at both the associate and full professor levels between 1981 and 1989. More recently, family medicine faculty members who were successfully promoted to associate professor had a mean of 7.6 peer-reviewed publications, and were first author on 5.5 publications. Only 43% had published at least one book chapter. While 64% had at least one training grant, only 44% had at least one research grant; 39% were the principal investigator on a research grant and 20% had federal research support (Zyzanski *et al*, 1996).

In a nine-year longitudinal study, Flocke *et al* (2004) found that baseline local mentoring and off-campus networking as measured by the Faculty Activities and Research Environment Survey (FARES) may be associated with promotion to associate professor. Similarly, baseline research activities, off-campus networking,

Table 9.3 Scholarship Clusters

	Publication		Presentation		Grants	
Principal Authorship	*Major Publications*	*Total Publications*	*Research Presentations*	*Other Presentations*	*Funding*	*Grants*
Number of invited publications	% Research publications	Total no. of publications	% Research presentations	Total no. of presentations	No. of funded grants	Total no. of grants
% Solo publications	(% Chapters)	No. of submissions	Research : non-research	No. of submissions	% Funded	No. of submissions
% First-author publications		No. of major publications		No. of plenary presentations	No. funded as principal investigator	No. of major grants
Research : non-research		No. of solo publications		No. of invited presentations		No. of grants as principal investigator
		No. of first-author publications		No. of conferences presented at		No. of research grants
		No. of journals published in				

( ) = Inverse association.

and scholarly habits were linked to attaining tenure among those faculty members remaining at the institution.

In addition to success rate, the speed of promotion depends upon publications. In a study among radiology faculty, "early promotion" was defined as under six years at the assistant professor level and under five years at the associate professor level. Those faculty receiving early promotion had more original (3.35 versus 1.82) and total publications (5.92 versus 2.85) as assistant professors than other radiology faculty. Those with early promotion also spent more time in administration (8.5 versus 4.6 hours). As associate professors, those receiving early promotion differed only in the number of original publications (4.03 versus 2.96). No differences in funding were found (Vydareny *et al*, 1999).

In addition, there are differences between clinician-educators and clinician-investigators. For clinician-educators, the most important performance aspects are teaching and clinical skills, mentoring, reputation and co-ordinating clerkship or curriculum development. At those institutions that required minimum levels of publications, clinician-investigators were expected to have more peer-reviewed publications than clinician-educators for promotion to associate professor (mean of 10.6 versus 5.7 publications) (Beasley *et al*, 1997).

But how do measures of publication, presentation, and grants interrelate, and what are the predictors for nomination and promotion at the associate and full professor levels? Do these predictors differ on the tenure versus non-tenure tracks? What are the predictors for receiving tenure on the tenure track?

Studies performed within our department over the past 15 years have revealed clusters of scholarship variables (*see* Table 9.3). Taking the three forms of scholarly productivity (publications, presentations, and grants) separately, publication variables fell into three factors:

- *principal authorship* included the number of solo publications, number of first-authored publications, number of invited publications, and the ratio of research to non-research publication
- *major publications* included the number of research publications, but was inversely related to the number of book chapters
- *total publications* included a variety of other publication variables.

Presentation variables clustered into *research presentation variables* and *other presentation variables*. Finally, grantmanship variables clustered into *funding variables* and *other grant variables*. Conversely, if these variables are not separated out by the form of scholarship they represent and include national service variables, a different pattern is seen. In this case, three factors result. One factor represents *national service* and includes involvement on national committees and hosting national conferences. Another factor includes invited presentations and having funded grants. Finally, a reputation factor is seen, which includes not only invited and other publications, but service as a journal reviewer and on editorial boards.

How do these different scholarship and service variables interact to lead to a faculty member being nominated for promotion and attaining promotion? Table 9.4 presents the results of such an analysis within one department of family medicine in an academic health center; although representing a single case study, there may be lessons for all departments. Although Beasley *et al* (1997) found that chairs of P&T committees indicate that clinician-educators are promoted based heavily upon their teaching and clinical activities, our study found very different results for non-tenure track faculty (which presumably includes the majority of clinician-educators). The departmental P&T committee was more likely to recommend promotion for faculty with plenary presentations but not funded grants. Publications were also important; major publications (research, chapters, reviews) versus others (editorials, letters, case reports, book reviews) differentiated between assistant and associate professors. Major publications predicted recommendations for promotion in assistant professors, but other publications predicted such recommendations for associate professors. Once nominated for promotion, the institution's P&T committee was less likely to award promotion to those faculty members currently involved in teaching, extra-departmental service, and patient care, but more likely to award promotion to those involved in grant activity since their last promotion or appointment.

Patterns among tenure track faculty are equally interesting. As expected, nomination for promotion relied upon publications, presentations, grants, and service as a national reviewer. In addition, nomination also depended upon current national service and local service. Although research presentations and national reviewing were important no matter what rank, successful promotion differed for assistant and associate professors. Assistant professors were successful if they served on and chaired committees, but were less successful with more presentations over the past three years and publications since being appointed. However, associate professors were successful based upon expected patterns. Associate professors were promoted with national service rather than university/state service or committee work. In addition, presentations in the past three years and recent publications were positive predictors of promotion.

Recommendations for tenure also depended heavily upon scholarly activity. Not only were cumulative publications, presentations, grants, and national reviewing important, but current national service, major publications, presentations as first presenter, and principal investigator on grants were as well. Nomination for tenure was also associated with external collaboration, administrative responsibilities as director, and university/state service. Once nominated for tenure, tenure was awarded to those faculty members serving on departmental committees, publishing as first authors, and making research (as opposed to plenary) presentations, but inversely related to the amount of grant awards received as principal investigator; institutional service was not a predictor. These results differ from those of Zyzanski *et al* (1996) who found that MDs successfully seeking tenure had more peer-reviewed publications, more than one book chapter, and more research and training grant support, and federal research funding.

The findings presented above emphasize the discrepancy between promotional criteria reportedly used by P&T committees and factors actually linked to promotion and tenure. How can this information be used by the research director to prepare faculty for promotion?

Preparing for Promotion

Although specific criteria for and recommendations about promotion may differ from institution to institution, the research director can recommend that certain general principles be followed. First, plan early; don't wait to prepare for promotion. Seek advice along the way from the chair, mentors, the departmental

Table 9.4 Correlates of Promotion/Tenure Nomination and Success

	Promotion	Tenure
Nomination		
Current Activity		
scholarship		% External collaboration (+)
publications	Total (+)	Total (+)
	Invited (+ACP)	Major (+)
		% Chapters (−)
		% Publications (+)
presentations	Invited (+)	First presenter (+)
	First presenter (+)	
	% First presenter conferences (−)	
grants	Total (+ACP)	% As primary investigator (+)
	As primary investigator (+ACP)	
service		
local	University/state service (+)	Division director (+)
	University committees (+)	University/state service (+)
	University committees chaired (+ACP)	Hospital committees (−)
	State committees chaired (+)	
national	National service (+)	National service (+)
	National committees (+ATP)	National committees (+)
	National committees chaired (+)	Reviewing activity (+)
	Reviewing activity (+)	
Cumulative Activity		
scholarship	Total publications (+)	Total publications (+)
	% Publications (+)	% Publications (+)
	Total presentations (+)	Total presentations (+)
	Total grants (+)	% Research presentations (−)
		Total grants (+)
		Grants as primary investigator (+)
service	Reviewing activity (+)	Conference reviewing (+)
		Journal reviewing (+)
Success		
Current Activity		
scholarship		
publications		Refereed (−)
		% First-author (+)
presentations		Total (−)
		% Research (+)
		Plenary (−)
		% First presenter conferences (+)
grants		Funded as primary investigator (−)
		$ Funding as primary investigator (−)
service	Total committees (+ATP, −ACP)	Departmental committees (+)
	Total committees chaired (+ATP, −ACP)	
	University/state service (−ACP)	
	National service (+ACP)	
	Reviewing activity (+)	
interval	Total publications since (−ATP, +ACP)	Research presentations (+)
scholarship	Publications in last 3 years (+ACP)	Non-research presentations (−)
	Presentations in last 3 years (−ATP, +ACP)	
	Research presentations (+)	

ATP: assistant professor; ACP: associate professor.

P&T committee. Have your record reviewed annually to provide you with feedback. Know the promotion criteria and process at your institution, and compare your record and curriculm vitae (CV) against others' CVs and against the records of faculty in other comparable clinical departments. Keep everything that could possibly impact your career, including annual reports of activity and evaluations, syllabi, citations and publications, reviews of your work, awards, instructional analyses, and unsolicited letters and commendations. Also, share developments with your chair. In general, quality is considered more important than quantity (American Geriatric Society Education Committee, 2002).

Scholarly activity (e.g. publications, presentations, grants) is the easiest to document. Reviewers on promotion and tenure committees are looking for evidence of sustained, independent activity, usually with a focus. Thus, you want to concentrate on publishable studies early in your career and reporting research that is current or resulted in dissemination. Although review committees do consider presentations at national meetings, service on dissertation or research review committees, and grant support, grant support without publication is not enough. The ultimate measure of research productivity is publications. Although research publications are the most valuable, scholarly review articles in peer-reviewed journals are also worthwhile. Case reports and letters-to-the-editor do not count for much. Book chapters can be valuable in areas where little research has been done (Kazerooni, 1997). Writing books is inadvisable until tenure is secured, due to the time investment. In which journals should you publish? Although the ultimate answer may be ''any journal that will publish your manuscript'', different journals do count differently (Beasley *et al*, 1997). Although *New England Journal of Medicine* and *JAMA* publications are most valued, family medicine faculty rarely publish there. Successful family medicine faculty have typically published in *Journal of Family Practice, Family Medicine,* and *Academic Medicine* (Gjerde *et al*, 1982; Gjerde, 1992). However, family medicine researchers often publish in non-family medicine journals (Katerndahl *et al*, 1998).

Teaching is scholarly when one writes about curricula, is an invited speaker, develops innovations, receives grant awards. Teaching documentation includes lecture and course responsibilities, continuing medical education (CME) presentations, role modeling, and development of innovative methods or media. Supervision and advising also count, especially if you can document the subsequent success of those you advised. Objective evidence of teaching excellence, such as student and peer evaluations, instructional analysis, and student scores on objective tests are highly valued (Beasley *et al*, 1997). Teaching awards serve as external recognition of excellence. Excellence in teaching based on peer review requires innovation.

When evaluating service, it is important to remember that service includes more than patient care or departmental administration; it also includes service to the institution, the community, and the discipline. But not all service is equally valued. Generally, service to the university counts more than service to the hospital. Committees differ in how they are valued; the admissions committee, the institutional review board, and the committee-on-committees are highly valued. For clinical service, clinical productivity and evaluations from peers and patients count (Beasley *et al*, 1997). In general, review committees look for the level of responsibility, committee work, consultations, key administrative duties, and review activities.

Most institutions are also concerned with national and international reputa-tion. Thus, external awards, invited presentations, solicitation of your input or consultation, and holding office in national organizations are strong evidence of reputation (Beasley *et al*, 1997). Generally, the evidence can be divided into direct and indirect evidence. Direct evidence includes invited publications and pre-sentations, appointments to review panels and editorial boards, reviews and citations of your work, elected or appointed offices in organizations, external awards, and grant contracts. Indirect evidence includes national presentations and publications, receipt of national grants, and service on national committees or review panels for which you volunteered. Generally, your reputation is assumed if you have enough publications and/or grants. Because your CV only documents invited publications and presentations that you deliver, you must save evidence of invitations that you decline so they can be included in your promotion package.

Finally, although the future of tenure may be in doubt, it is still a measure of academic success. Tenure is typically based upon vaguely defined criteria. In addition to qualities desirable in faculty, P&T committees are looking for value to the institution through collaboration across departments, achievement congruent with the institution's mission, or a unique institutional role. They are also looking for sustained performance, which predicts ongoing performance. Thus, waiting until just before being reviewed to produce ("tenure-busting") is not valued. The issue of sustained performance has become enough of a concern that many institutions now require periodic post-tenure review.

Thus, there are a few basic rules to ensuring that a faculty member's career is constantly moving toward promotion. First, keep track of every professional activity as it happens; don't rely upon memory. Teaching, service, and research can reinforce each other if there is a focus to your activities. Publication is the most valued activity and must be continuously pursued. Thus, the goal is to have an ongoing stream of manuscripts in preparation and review; resubmit manu-scripts whenever possible. Collaboration can help one's career. Not only can senior collaborators complement a junior's skills, but they can promote one's career in numerous ways. Finally, get feedback often and examine the CVs of other successful faculty. Promotion does not just happen; it goes to the diligent and prepared. Just prior to being recommended for promotion, certain strategies are advised. First, avoid a last minute drop-off in scholarly productivity. Finish old projects before starting new ones. Consider where and when to submit manu-scripts; a manuscript in press with a second-tier journal counts more than a manuscript under review at a first-tier journal. Avoid political arguments that may lead to animosity among members of the P&T committee. Finally, avoid new teaching assignments as tenure review draws near, because they increase work-load and often result in poor evaluations until the "bugs" are worked out.

Evidence for Promotion

Curriculum Vitae

The CV is the written representation of your professional career and, as such, must be complete. Thus, everything must be documented in the format required by the institution. There is no place for modesty in one's CV. Second, the CV must be understandable to its intended audience – the institutional P&T committee. Thus, entries may need to be annotated so that their significance can be appreciated. Finally, the CV must be readable. Thus, an adequate font (e.g. 12-point), adequate margins, and appropriate spacing within and between entries must be used.

Documentation of research scholarship not only includes publications, presentations, and funding, but should also include evidence of peer review. Thus, internal review and external letters can show the significance of one's scholarship as well as its impact. Ultimately, citations are evidence of the impact of work (Aday and Quill, 2000). In addition, recent suggestions have been proposed for documenting collaboration on research. If such collaboration is listed on a CV, entries should include the name of the project's principal investigator and one's role on the project (Davies *et al*, 1996).

Documentation of teaching should include *all* teaching activities. However, recurrent lectures or one-on-one precepting should be presented as recurrent activities, rather than listed individually each time they occur. Unnecessary redundancy on a CV gives the appearance of "padding". In addition to teaching activities, one needs to include media and software prepared, materials, innovative methods, and evaluation activities as well. It is also appropriate to list formal study designed to improve teaching and administrative skills.

Finally, when documenting service, remember to include all areas of service from the discipline to the community. Service is the area most likely to need clarification for the P&T committee to appreciate. Therefore, annotation may be necessary to explain the duties and responsibilities of administrative positions or committee assignments.

Portfolios

Portfolios summarize faculty activity in a particular area. Although typically used to document teaching activity, portfolios can also document research and service. Table 9.5 presents the categories included within portfolios and how each category is applied to teaching, research, and service. Although all of the categories are valuable for promotional purposes, the categories under "Promotion" deal with evidence of productivity. Thus, for teaching, this means modules and courses developed as well as learner performance. For research, this means research instruments developed and citations of one's work. For service, this means service-related materials developed and evidence of the impact of service. "Skills" describes activities in teaching, research, and service. Teaching portfolios document the current status of advisees, and education-related committees and leadership. In addition, education-related scholarship and honors are documented. For research, performance of protégés, and research-related committees and leadership are included. In addition, research-related scholarship and honors are documented. For service, performance of subordinates, and service-related committees and leadership is included. In addition, service-related scholarship and honors are documented.

Finally, under "Faculty development", a 1–2 page statement of philosophy concerning outcomes, roles, and responsibilities in education, research, and service is included. In addition, courses taken to improve teaching, research, or

Table 9.5 Contents of Teaching, Research, and Service Portfolios

Category	Teaching	Research	Service
Promotion			
Development	Modules/courses	Instruments	Materials
Impact	Learner performance	Citations	Service impact
Skills	Teaching activities	Research activities	Service activities
Advisor	Advisees' performance	Protégés' performance	Subordinates' performance
Administration	Leadership/service positions	Leadership/service positions	Leadership/service positions
Scholarship	Publications, presentations, grants	Publications, presentations, grants	Publications, presentations, grants
Honors	Recognition	Recognition	Recognition
Faculty development			
Philosophy	Education	Scholarship	Service
Continuing education	Activities	Activities	Activities
Long-term goals and strategies	Goals with timeline	Goals with timeline	Goals with timeline

clinical/administrative skills are listed. Finally, long-term goals in each are presented along with the strategies used to achieve those goals and a timeline.

Letters-of-Support

Letters-of-support are generally critical to a promotion package. Although internal letters (from the chair, administrators, and collaborators) can clarify relevant issues that are unique to the faculty member or his/her discipline, generally it is the external letters that are the most important. In fact, certain characteristics can only be documented through letters. External letters can document the quality of the work, and one's expertise and authority within an area. Letters document an emerging or established reputation. Finally, external letters allow their writers to emphasize one's "promotability" at their institutions. But, because external letters can be so important, one must choose the people who write them carefully. First, select people at institutions of equivalent or higher prestige, but ensuring that they understand the standards at your institution. Choose people of higher rank with at least some full professors. If part of a research team, only ask one member of the team for a letter-of-support, preferably the principal investigator. Finally, know who selects the letters that will be included in the package. If all letters received are included, then one needs to select people who will uniformly give strong endorsements. On the other hand, if the chair can select letters to be included from those received, there is less concern that one may inadvertently receive a poor letter that could sabotage the package.

Personal Statement

Generally, personal statements are unnecessary; the CV and letters speak for themselves. But there are circumstances when this is not true and a personal statement may prevent the P&T committee from misreading the record. The personal statement is most helpful when a CV *appears* to show a decline in productivity for no obvious reason. In this case, it is critical that this impression is exposed as incorrect or the chances for promotion drop. The typical situation is where research productivity has dropped due to administrative responsibilities or a change in research focus. In the first case, the statement needs to clarify the administrative burden that produced this decline; in the second case, the statement needs to document this shift and discuss the importance of this new focus (Aday and Quill, 2000). Finally, a personal statement can be helpful if it may appear that the scholarship is unfocused. As family physicians, we can approach this in two ways. First, one can argue that, as a generalist, one should not be expected to focus. Although this strategy can work, generally a focus is desirable even for generalists. The second approach is to pull disparate works together through a common thread. Here, after reviewing past accomplishments, one needs to place one's research into a unified framework within the discipline. Finally, one should discuss one's goals and demonstrate how future work will build on past accomplishments.

Synthesis

Helping your faculty to achieve professional success through promotion and tenure can be extremely rewarding. Achieving promotability is an active process that cannot be left to the last minute, but rather must be engineered as soon as the faculty member is appointed or receives their first promotion. Knowing what is required for promotion or tenure should guide decisions about professional activities. The development of habits of ongoing documentation is critical. In addition, following proven guidelines for enhancing promotability will facilitate, and shorten the process for promotion and tenure.

As research director, it is your responsibility to facilitate this process by ensuring certain developments. First, a departmental P&T committee should be appointed to review faculty CVs on an annual basis. Second, faculty development activities must include discussions of the P&T process and criteria. Third, mentors need to address promotion and tenure issues with their protégés. Finally, faculty success should be celebrated throughout the department.

Chapter 10

Planning Research Careers

Vignette

J.O. was finishing his residency and planning on a career in academia. He knew that he should look for a research fellowship first and had already established a mentoring relationship with one of his faculty members. His chair was wanting him to join the faculty after his fellowship, but he wasn't sure whether this was the right department for his research career. On the advice of his mentor, he sat down and identified his five-year career goals and the opportunities that would be available to him in this department. At this point in time, his goals and the department's resources didn't appear to be a good match so he decided to "keep his options open".

Within a discipline, most research is the work of a few researchers. For example, in clinical laboratory science, 10% of the faculty produces more than half of the scholarly activity. In particular, these 10% contribute 49% of the national presentations, 54% of the research publications, 57% of the funded grants, and 70% of the international presentations (Waller *et al*, 1999). Pathman *et al* (2005) found that 7% of family medicine researchers authored 51% of the research articles. How does a faculty member plan to become one of these highly productive researchers?

Who is a Productive Researcher?

Demographically, males tend to publish more often (Barnett *et al*, 1998) and secure funding more often (Ferrer and Katerndahl, 2002) than do females; Caucasians publish more often than minority faculty members (Barnett *et al*, 1998). The relationship between marital status and productivity is less clear. Although Barnett *et al* (1998) found no relationship between publications and either marital status or parenting, Ferrer and Katerndahl (2002) found that, when adjusted for gender, single faculty members published less, while separated/divorced faculty members made fewer national presentations. In addition, the number of children at home was a positive predictor of five-year publications and presentations.

Research experience during medical school, class rank, and graduating Alpha Omega Alpha were predictors of faculty citations (Brancati *et al*, 1992). Although faculty rank is correlated with increasing publications, presentations, and funding (Waller *et al*, 1999), Ferrer and Katerndahl (2002) found a relationship only between associate/full professorship and five-year presentations. However, seniority was inversely related to current publications (Bartle *et al*, 2000).

Degree status is important. Waller *et al* (1999) found that clinical laboratory faculty with a PhD produced more publications, presentations, and funded grants than those with only a masters' degree. Ferrer and Katerndahl (2002) showed that MDs had fewer five-year funded grants, but PhDs and MDs with an advanced degree published more. Being on the tenure track was a predictor of five-year funding (Ferrer and Katerndahl, 2002).

Perhaps most important is motivation. Barnett *et al* (1998) found that intrinsic motivation (personal drive to conduct research) was a positive predictor, but extrinsic motivation (external rewards from research) was a negative predictor of publications. In fact, many of the previously reported correlates of productivity may actually reflect intrinsic motivation. Ultimately, the lack of this internal motivation to pursue research may be why generalists consistently report lower levels of scholarly productivity.

Training

A productive primary care research career begins with a period of structured training, generally in a fellowship setting. This experience should address skill development and instill professional identity and values. This training period must include access to advisors (Bland and Schmitz, 1986). This training period should also include two research experiences. It should feature a research apprenticeship under senior researchers, and it should include independent research experience in an area, encouraging the novice to begin to develop a track record in a field of study (Mainous, 2003). But fellowship alone is not a guarantee of early success. National Research Service Award (NRSA) fellows often are not productive; only 13% publish more than one article per year and only 42% are principal investigators on grants early in their careers (Curtis *et al*, 2003).

Early Career

When negotiating their first faculty appointment, new faculty should observe certain principles to avoid being taken for granted and having their research time usurped by teaching and clinical duties. First, they should match their position to the department's needs while ensuring that what they do well will be rewarded. Second, new faculty should outline an agenda for their career and establish with the chair a common definition for "success". Third, they need to position themselves within the department so that they will be considered "unique" in some way. Finally, new faculty must ensure that they have adequate resources, including mentors (Goldman, 1991). A correct, mutually rewarding initial appointment can facilitate the researcher's early career, so important to a productive faculty life.

A researcher's career is often determined by the first 3–5 years (Goldman, 1991; Hollenberg, 1992). During those first years, the researcher must have a clear job description and assured income. In addition, he/she needs opportunities for growth such as a productive environment, and research and travel support. The novice researcher must also have career-coaching opportunities such as periodic review and counseling (Hollenberg, 1992). This agrees with the findings of Bland and Schmitz (1986) that researchers early in their careers need mentoring with limited autonomy. In addition, ongoing support is critical to the continued productivity of faculty (Bland and Schmitz, 1986). In fact, the level of funding a department receives under the HRSA Academic Administrative Units grant program predicts 16% of the variance in per faculty publications (Wagner *et al*, 1994).

A sufficient amount of time must be dedicated to research, preferably at least 40% (Bland and Schmitz, 1986). Dedicated time for scholarship is predictive of the number of publications among faculty (Barnett *et al*, 1998). Many academic faculty have no dedicated research time (Waller *et al*, 1999). Hueston (1993a) found that three variables predicted having at least 10% of time dedicated to research – fellowship experience, years in academia, and belonging to a university-based family medicine department. Among clinical laboratory science faculty members, certain faculty characteristics correlate with the balance between research and teaching time. Teaching hours progressively decrease with increasing rank; conversely, research time increases as faculty move from assistant to associate professor. While non-tenure track faculty have less research time, tenure track faculty report that their research time drops from 9.8 hours per week to 5.7 hours when they receive tenure; their teaching hours also drop from 23.4 to 20.0 hours (Waller *et al*, 1999). It is unclear whether these decreases are mandated by department chairs, reflect increasing administrative duties, or reflect decreased faculty commitment to productivity once tenure is secured.

Finally, the balance between focus and variety is important. Baldwin (1983) found that faculty with varied careers were more productive over time. However, there are advantages to focusing scholarly efforts. First, having a focus allows us to develop personal expertise, which in turn can serve as a source of referrals and prevent "burnout". Second, many institutional promotion and tenure committees expect to see such a focus at the professor level. For some, the department may be able to successfully argue that, as a generalist, a focus is inappropriate. Finally, a focus helps to build a curriculum vitae (CV), because the research, teaching, and service tend to reinforce each other, and build a reputation. Choosing a focus must rest upon personal interest. However, consider the importance of the focus to primary care, the state of the literature, the availability of collaborators and mentors, and the availability of funding. Once a focus for scholarly work has been selected, one must immerse oneself continuously in the content and methodological literature. Conferences related to the focus should be attended to establish professional networks. One must begin communicating with national audiences to build a reputation through conference presentations and publication of reviews and case reports. Finally, one must begin to contribute to the research literature. Ultimately, a focus will provide numerous professional benefits.

Early in a research career, a faculty member needs to correctly negotiate his/her position including sufficient research time with limited autonomy, and work toward early productivity in terms of publications and grants. Pursuing a professional focus early will build your CV and facilitate promotion.

Planning

Steps in Career Planning

Productive academic careers don't just happen; they are the products of planning and constant attention (*see* Box 10.1). Perhaps the most important part of planning is the identification of career goals. Where do you want to be in five or ten years? What do you want to accomplish and what position do you want? The first step in career planning is to identify your goals and timetable for achievement. Appendix 1 includes instruments to assist in this process. Before proceeding, evaluate the feasibility of the goals and timeframe. For example, if the goals include becoming a dean and a National Institutes of Health (NIH)-supported researcher, they are probably mutually exclusive unless delegated to different timeframes.

Box 10.1 Steps in Career Planning

1. Identify goals and timeline
2. Assess status and potential
   - Current status
   - Research activity
   - Predicted research success
   - Collaborators and mentors
3. Assess access to resources
4. Self-evaluation

Once the goals are identified, current status must be assessed using a job activity analysis (*see* Appendix 1). One lists key academic activities and the time spent on each. Then, strengths and weaknesses are appraised as well as needs related to each activity. Finally, each activity is rated as to the value and satisfaction to the department and oneself. This exercise allows critical appraisal of time spent, and its value both personally and to the department. It also allows recognition of activities in which there is a discrepancy in value between personal value and value to the department. Do these activities help in achieving the long-term goals? Are there activities of little value to both oneself and the department, which could be eliminated? Second, focusing on a research career, what is one's current research activity? Completing an instrument such as the one in Appendix 1 can help in this assessment. To evaluate personal current research activity, ask oneself whether there is a balance between research and non-research scholarly activity. Is there some involvement in grant writing? Is there involvement in multiple studies at different stages? Are articles being published at a rate of at least two publications per year? Finally, the assessment of current status should include an estimation of predicted success. The Faculty Activities and Research Environment Survey (FARES) can provide scores in the areas of local mentoring, research activity, networking, and scholarly habits (*see* Appendix 1). If the sum of the research activity and scholarly habits scores is at least 7, this is predictive of future research success, defined as receipt of funding and publication of at least two papers per year. Finally, list the collaborators and mentors with whom one currently works departmentally, institutionally, and externally. Indicate their expertise or area of mentorship (*see* Appendix 1).

Once current status is assessed, it is time to critically evaluate potential access to resources departmentally and institutionally. Start by listing potential collaborators and mentors, and in what area they could help (*see* Appendix 1). Indicate what opportunities are available for advanced training and their time commitment. Identify what institutional facilities are available and their level of support. What human and material resources are available in the department? Identify departmental and institutional opportunities for faculty development and evaluation. Finally, list the availability of grant support locally.

At this point, one has identified where one wants to go, where one currently is, and what resources are available. Synthesizing this wealth of information can lead to identifying the skills and support needed to achieve the goals. Prioritization of these goals can help in making some hard decisions. For example, can one achieve the most important goals at the current institution?

Finally, an ongoing process of self-evaluation is critical to keep one on track. Although this should include self-evaluation, it should also include evaluation by the mentor and chair. This appraisal should include assessment of personal growth, new development, and effectiveness in current activities.

Stages in a Career

Early in an academic career, issues include time constraints, skill development, role ambiguity, and inexperience (*see* Box 10.2). Some of these issues can be addressed through an orientation program and a written job description. In addition, identification of a mentor and participation in regular faculty evaluation can help. Time must be allocated and protected for research and writing. Skill development through faculty development and fellowship training is essential. As a researcher, necessary skills include co-ordination and project management skills, in addition to the research, statistical, presentation, and writing skills integral to the research endeavor. Finally, a research focus should be sought, even among generalists.

Box 10.2 Career Issues and Career Stage

Early Career
- Time constraints
- Skill development
- Role ambiguity
- Inexperience
- Choosing research focus

Mid-Career
- Recognition
- Advancement
- Expectations of colleagues
- Exploration of new career opportunities
- Leadership

Late Career
- Uncertainty about the future
- Possible stagnation
- Uncertainty about value of contribution

Once established, a career enters a period of integration. The mid-career issues revolve around seeking recognition and advancement, increased expectations of colleagues, and exploration of new career opportunities. Skill development may focus on advanced research skills, and the development and use of theory. These issues lead to increased leadership activity, advanced training, involvement in external activities and organizations, and service as a mentor to others.

Finally, at a senior stage, when recognized as a leader and expert, one is faced with internal challenges such as uncertainty about the future and the value of one's contribution, and the specter of stagnation. Methods for dealing with these challenges focus on diversification, and may include increased local leadership and/or greater external involvement, such as editorships, sabbaticals, and consultations. Development of a new area of focus or innovative research methods is another approach to these challenges.

Synthesis

As a faculty member, the message is "Planning, planning, and planning!" Career success is based on planning, and that career planning is an active, ongoing process. Without goals, one doesn't know how to proceed and what to evaluate. Achievement comes from setting benchmarks and meeting them. But a career does not unfold in a vacuum; it is a product of relationships, and the management of time and resources.

As research director, one must constantly attend to the career status of the faculty, aware of their goals and commitments, seeking opportunities that will help them in their career development. Although the development and success of faculty is rightly the chair's responsibility, the demands of being chair often necessitate the delegation of responsibility to others. The research director must assume this responsibility, promoting career development through mentorship, faculty development, and input from the departmental promotion and tenure committee.

Unfortunately, the research director cannot afford to focus upon individual researcher development alone. He/she is responsible for *departmental* productivity. It is possible to have productive researchers who create disharmony within the department and compromise group productivity. In addition, individual development can be approached through group development activities. Section III addresses promotion of departmental scholarship.

Section III

Promoting Research in the Department

## Chapter 11

Developing Culture

Vignette

The chair was the only one enthusiastic about establishing a research program within the department. He had given her free rein; he wanted her to get the research going and was willing to support her in any way he could to create a "culture of inquiry". But creating a new culture would be a challenge! K.N. decided to start by focusing on visible cues. She strategically posted banners reminding faculty of the departmental research goals. She organized faculty meeting research rituals, such as lighting candles for submitted grants. She recognized individual faculty members monthly with scholar awards during Grand Rounds presentations. Most faculty enjoyed these lighthearted activities and, slowly but steadily, research became an acceptable and frequent topic of conversation.

As important as developing research skills among individual faculty may be, the research director's primary responsibility is to the scholarly productivity of the department or residency program as a whole. But to do this in a previously non-productive environment, the departmental culture must be changed and, thus, the research director must have the support of the chair. As of 1994, family medicine chairs were rating the importance to the discipline of research, non-research scholarship, and fellowship training as seventh, eighth, and ninth respectively out of nine possible factors (Katerndahl, 1994). These dismal ratings may reflect the lack of research training and experience among senior chairs. In 1992, only 8% of chairs over 50 years of age had training in conducting research and only 18% had any research experience. These statistics were not much better among chairs aged under 50 years; although 45% did have research training, still only 18% had research experience (Murata *et al*, 1992). The fact that a department or residency has a faculty member designated as research director may reflect support for research, but it may also reflect only tacit support.

Support is critical if you are to create a culture that values research. Such a culture is essential. That "culture of inquiry" is vital to the future rigor of our discipline (Dickinson *et al*, 2000; Stange *et al*, 2001; Katerndahl *et al*, 2002). Family medicine research in research-intense institutions leads to more funded grants than that in less intense institutions, even when controlling for faculty size. Such research-intense institutions have more faculty, more faculty on research tracks, and more support staff. This emphasizes the need for a critical mass of researchers, and for research to be perceived as a priority (Mainous *et al*, 2000). Of the 15 factors that Eisenberg (1986) identified for success of primary care researchers (*see* Box 11.1), four reflect the setting or support of the chair. In addition to chair support and an academic research setting, he stressed the need for available collaborators and experienced researchers. Taken a step further, Page (1976) stated that the environment was more important to research productivity than was funding. His vision emphasized the need for leadership, recruitment, standards, and encouragement if the appropriate research environment is to be created (*see* Box 11.2). How does such a vision get translated into the development of a departmental research environment?

Box 11.1 Factors for Success (Adapted from Eisenberg, 1986)

1. Hard work
2. Conceptualizing ideas
3. Experience on project with mentors
4. Recognize important problems
5. Experience with independent research design
6. Availability of experienced researchers
7. Research knowledge
8. Chair supportive of research
9. Availability of collaborators
10. Training in methods
11. Protected time
12. Operationalizing problems
13. Academic research setting
14. Training that encourages/demands research
15. Mentors

Box 11.2 Encouraging a Research Environment (Adapted from Page, 1976)

1. Leadership with reason and advice
2. Selection of people dedicated primarily to research
3. Selection of research problems acceptable to investigators
4. Encouragement of intellectual competition
5. High standards and open communication
6. Active participation in research by leader
7. Advancement based on scientific achievement
8. Laboratories built on the needs of investigators
9. Encouragement of co-operation and mutual work
10. Pursuit of research with and without teaching duties
11. Emphasis on integrity and responsibility
12. Encouragement of open-mindedness and confidence to undertake new projects

---

Departmental Research Environment

In their review of the literature, Bland and Ruffin (1992) identified 12 consistent environmental characteristics in productive research units. Keeping these in mind, the research director has a framework for building a productive environment (Bland *et al*, 2005).

Clear Goals

The department needs clear research goals that serve a co-ordinating function. Goals should be based upon faculty strengths, societal needs, and funding opportunities. Such goals provide direction and can assist in making difficult decisions about the use of resources. Thus, if one of the departmental goals is to promote the department's reputation for scholarship, then funding for a scientific editor would be protected even during a time of financial stress.

Research Emphasis

Research should *not* be merely a third wheel in the department, stepchild to teaching and clinical service. Research needs to be an equal partner if the environment is to be truly supportive and ultimately productive. Thus, when the department opens a new ambulatory clinic, faculty time to staff the clinic is taken equally from teaching, clinical, and scholarly activities.

Distinctive Culture

Although each department has a culture distinctive to it, that culture needs to include research as part of its identity. Without that research culture, research will never be equal to the other missions of the department. Culture is built through communication, faculty development, recruitment of faculty, and peer modeling. Thus, scholarly rituals become part of the departmental milieu.

Positive Group Environment

The group attitude is critical to productivity. If members do not look forward to conducting their research, feel undervalued, and hesitate to collaborate with their colleagues, the often-draining endeavor called "research" becomes a chore, and productivity suffers. Thus, visible celebration of scholarly success should be a regular departmental activity.

Assertive Participative Governance

Faculty must feel that they play a role in the governance and decision making in the department. As intelligent, creative researchers, their opinions should be valued and be important in any decisions related to research. Thus, when the departmental budget is suddenly cut, *all* departmental faculty should actively participate in the decisions and budget planning that results.

Decentralized Organization

As an extension of participative governance, decision making within the department should be decentralized so that the department can respond creatively and quickly to problems and opportunities. If governance indeed rests with its members, there is no need for centralization of authority. Thus, productive research departments are not top-down organizations; they recognize the decision-making abilities of its division directors and individual faculty members.

Frequent Communication

Decisions and exploitation of opportunities can only be made efficiently if information is readily disseminated. Frequent communication is essential in productive environments. Thus, when the Agency for Healthcare Research and Quality (AHRQ) releases a new program announcement in health services research, the news is rapidly disseminated throughout the research division.

Accessible Resources

As mentioned above, the availability of resources, especially human resources, is vital to a productive research environment. Little can be achieved without pilot funding, access to computers and software, and interaction with collaborators and mentors. Thus, the research director must be able to quickly secure research assistant time to be dedicated to an investigator's pilot work prior to R01 submission.

Sufficient Size, Age, and Diversity

A critical mass of investigators is necessary for the establishment of a research culture, exchange of ideas, and availability of collaborators. The age of the research unit brings reputation and maturity, which open opportunities, and demographic and academic diversity brings new ideas and a wealth of skills. Thus, the research director wants to build a seasoned research unit with a wealth of both senior and junior faculty, with both MD and PhD faculty, with both quantitative and qualitative research skills.

Appropriate Rewards

Although we often focus upon financial rewards, non-financial rewards can be as effective in terms of creating a positive group environment and a sense of individual worth. Public acknowledgment of accomplishments may yield just as much as a financial bonus. Thus, departments should annually celebrate promotions and awards, funding, and publications.

Concentration on Recruitment and Selection

Because productive researchers are typically on "auto-pilot" and primarily need support and resources, the key to a productive department is having productive members. Thus, recruitment and selection of researchers who are currently productive or have the potential for productivity are essential. Recruitment criteria should include not only motivation, experience and excellence in research, but also collaboration, teaching skills, and goodness-of-fit with the department. The recruitment process should include active researchers within the institution, who may serve as collaborators with the faculty member being recruited, even if they are appointed in other departments.

Leadership with Research Experience

Leaders without research experience lack a true understanding of the demands of conducting research and the resources required. In addition, for decisions to be supported by the researchers, the leader must have the research credentials to be recognized as authoritative. The lack of research skills and experience among chairs may represent a barrier to departmental productivity. Although this can be dealt with via a credible research director, often the research director is inexperienced in research and administration, or lacks any true authority; this is another reason why the research director must be an established investigator. Thus, leaders need to be research oriented and be scholars themselves. In fact, it is the leader who is often responsible for the other characteristics, such as departmental goals, management of resources, participatory governance and identification of opportunities.

Chairs and research directors can use this information to build a productive research environment. Although leadership training may be necessary to implement participative governance, most of these characteristics can be addressed by simply attending to them. Do these concepts apply in the more resource-poor environments of residency programs?

Residency Research Environment

To facilitate the development of a research environment within a residency program, you must not only define "research" (and scholarship) broadly, but also foster an attitude of critical inquiry and value for research. You must encourage residents' participation in research, and then provide the tools and resources necessary to accomplish it. Finally, you must offer residents the opportunity to present their results (Geyman, 1977). Residencies that successfully create a research culture in residency usually have a research curriculum that begins early in training. In addition, time and funding for research is available, and faculty are actively involved (DeHaven *et al*, 1998). These recommendations were supported by Kuzel (1984) who found that program policy and faculty research activity predicted resident research, and that lack of resident and faculty research time were strong inhibitory factors.

Whether to require resident involvement in research is still hotly debated. Most faculty would probably recommend that, if required, any form of scholarship would be acceptable. In 1980, 15% of family medicine residencies required research, while 64% encouraged it (Wilson and Redman, 1980); in 1984, 15% of Illinois residencies required research, while 30% encouraged it (Kuzel and Piotrowski, 1984). In 1997, 29% of programs required a research project of residents (DeHaven *et al*, 1997) and, by 2002, 49% required a research project (Neale, 2002). By contrast, 43% of rehabilitation residencies in 1994 required residents to do research, and 8% had a mandatory research rotation (Taniguchi and Johnson, 1994); 57% of physiatric residencies had a research requirement (Blake *et al*, 1994). In 1996, 97% of internal medicine residencies expected residents to participate in scholarly activity and 55–62% of their third-year residents were involved in research activity (*see* Table 11.1). Internal medicine residents at university programs were more likely to indicate that curiosity rather than mandate was their reason for participation in research (Alguire *et al*, 1996). Among rehabilitation residencies, only a research requirement was associated with residents submitting abstracts for presentation or manuscripts for publication (Taniguchi and Johnson, 1994), while among physiatric residencies, a research curriculum, faculty and resident guidelines about mentorship, and an external mentor predicted resident productivity (Blake *et al*, 1994). The reasons for family medicine residencies not requiring resident participation in research usually include inadequate numbers and experience of faculty, or inadequate resources. Only 26% of programs indicated that their reason for not requiring research was related to a lack of resident interest (Wilson and Redman, 1980). University and non-university internal medicine residencies differ in their barriers to resident research; university programs more often indicate that lack of resident time is a barrier, while non-university programs cite the lack of faculty time, role models, and faculty interest as important (Alguire *et al*, 1996).

Table 11.1 Proportions (%) of Residencies Requiring Research Based on Specialty

Specialty	1980	1984	1994	1996	1997	2002
Family medicine	15	15[a]			29	49
Rehabilitation medicine			43			
Physiatry			57			
Internal medicine				97		

[a] Illinois Residencies.

DeHaven *et al* (1998) feel not only that the required research projects are important to creating a research culture, but also that a research curriculum, begun early, is necessary. Research activities should have high visibility and be seen as part of evidence-based medicine. A research committee should co-ordinate such research activities. Of the programs that required research, half (46%) had 6–10 faculty, while most encouraged faculty research (71%) and had a research curriculum for residents (69%). Although enforcement is often not emphasized (54%), and annual promotion is not linked to research progress (78%), residents usually select their topic based on interest (85%), but faculty often must approve the topic (52%). Ultimately, 44% of programs require residents to present results at a research day, and such a presentation often (48%) serves as the criterion for completion of the project (Neale, 2002).

A variety of strategies need to be employed if a program is serious about resident research, in addition to the obvious emphasis on evidence-based medicine with its journal clubs and value assigned to research. Once faculty research is established, resident skill-building opportunities such as research grand rounds, and involvement in research development conferences are needed. Questions arising during patient care provide an opportunity for a teachable ''researchable'' moment and interest in research. Another method for stimulating resident interest in research might involve the requirement of residents to rotate through practices involved in practice-based research. A resident research requirement is the best way to ensure that all residents get exposed to the possibilities that research offers, even if this is conducted as a group project. But such a research requirement means that resources must be provided. In addition to computer access, pilot funds, and research assistants, residents must have sufficient time available to commit to research; longitudinal time dedicated to research is vital, supplemented by elective opportunities. In addition to a high-profile annual departmental research conference at which residents present their research, travel funds should be available for residents to present at national meetings. Finally, for those residents with an interest in research, the residency should consider developing a research track designed to nurture this interest, perhaps including travel funds to attend the North American Primary Care Research Group (NAPCRG) annual meeting.

Resident research should not be an afterthought, supported with little more than words and producing little more than resident angst. Wilson and Redman (1980) found that, compared to programs only encouraging research, programs that required research had more residents present their results (79% versus 40%) and submit written reports (69% versus 34%), although no difference in external dissemination was found. Internal medicine residents felt that research projects (26%) as well as publications and presentations (21%) are important (Alguire *et al*, 1996). Curtis (1980) suggested that, while research courses and participation in research projects were the strategies for teaching residents about research, publications, self-esteem, and opportunities to present results were their rewards.

Medical Student Research

Part of developing a research culture may include promoting medical student research within the department. Premedical major is not related to student research (Schaad *et al*, 1984). Curtis (1980) suggested that, while electives and assistantships are the strategies for teaching students about research, funding and opportunities to present results are their rewards. The University of Colorado's program included the implementation of a family medicine scholars' program, as well as identification of faculty mentors, setting research agendas geared to student schedules, co-ordination with predoctoral activities, and provision of research funds. This program increased the number of students involved in research from 8 in 1990–91 to 30 in 1996–97, with commensurate increases in the number of presentation submissions from 0 to 9 and of publication submissions from 0 to 5 (Gonzales *et al*, 1998). Thus, student research as well as that of faculty and residents can be fostered.

Synthesis

Ultimately, whether promoting research in departments or residencies, the first and key step to success is cultural change. But cultural change does not come easy . . . or cheap. Departments and residencies must be willing to invest time and money into the effort, and be willing to suffer through the inevitable period of discontent and resistance. Many of the strategies designed to build the culture are free. They include such activities as verbalized expectations, constant and consistent reminders, and high-profile messages, such as resources committed to conferences and presentations.

However, two critical pieces are difficult to establish and maintain. Trust must exist for faculty to share ideas, work in synergistic teams, or open themselves to critique of their designs, grant proposals, and manuscripts. Faculty must feel respected and secure in the knowledge that they will not be ridiculed or their position compromised. Second, a productive environment is an energetic environment. Investigators must feel energized by their investigations, feeding on each other's excitement, until the creative energy is palpable. For this reason, researchers must be in close proximity to each other, sharing common space. Ultimately, though, it is the research director's responsibility to stoke the excitement, to keep the research unit charged. Thus, success or failure in research promotion within a department or residency is a matter of commitment on behalf of its leadership . . . including that of its research director.

## Chapter 12

Stages of Departmental Research Development

Vignette

K.N. had been successful in establishing a productive research program; the department was indeed recognized for its research. The problem was that the research consisted of numerous small, unrelated (and largely unfunded) studies. It was time to focus on turning the research program into a sustainable research unit, producing high-impact work. K.N. began by looking at ways to bring the various research collaborations together under a common theme, working toward a group of R01-funded projects that could serve as the core for a research center. At their research retreat, the investigators began by focusing on the long-term departmental research goals and themes.

The successful inculcation of research into departmental activities requires a change in culture. Family medicine departments are rarely founded with research recognized as a core mission. Typically, the departmental foundation consists of teaching and clinical care. Only after the department matures and seeks an equal footing with other institutional departments does research become a priority. By that time, a culture focused on teaching and clinical care is well established. For research to become an equal partner at that point requires a change in culture.

Such a change in academic culture means that its members must change their attitudes and beliefs, a slow resisted process. This can only happen with commitment from the chair, energy and enthusiasm from the research director, and constant attention to promoting the message. Not only must members be reminded of the value of research, but reminders must occur continuously. Leaders must consistently convey the message that research is a core mission, is valued by academic family physicians, and is expected of departmental faculty. As we discuss possible departmental activities designed to promote research, remember that the value of any activity may rest more on its impact in changing culture than its more obvious intent. Thus, faculty development activities themselves may do little to stimulate research productivity, but the fact that they occur and are attended by the majority of faculty may go a long way to remolding the departmental culture into one that values and expects scholarship.

The Department of Family and Community Medicine at the University of Missouri has classified research programs into five stages. Aside from programs with no research activity, programs can be classified as those with emerging, entrepreneurial, or sustainable research. Eventually, programs may come to the stage of replication of research. Let us begin by looking at the emergence of research.

Developing Research *de novo*

Departments that lack a history of scholarship pose the greatest challenge. Although faculty in such departments may recognize the need for research in the discipline, they often fail to accept their role in producing that research or deem it impossible to do. Making research seem possible begins by redefining "research" to include non-research scholarship such as reviews and case studies. Of the 12 environmental characteristics listed in Chapter 11, seven are most critical. These include positive group environment, concentration on recruitment and selection, frequent communication, accessible resources (especially mentors), and sufficient size, age, and diversity (especially collaborators). But, most critical are clear goals and leadership with research experience (Bland *et al*, 2005.

If we accept that scholarship is the product of motivation and capacity built on need (*see* Figure 12.1), then establishing a need or sense of urgency is the first step. A shared vision must be created and include departmental research goals as well as a research component to the departmental mission statement. Harris *et al* (2003) suggest that the next step is to form a coalition of educators and champions to guide the process. This coalition creates the vision and plan, including setting criteria and rewards, and recognizing key people. The coalition then communicates this vision to the department. Although a key individual or individuals must develop the plan, I recommend involving the entire faculty in creating the research vision to encourage "buy-in". No plan can succeed, however, without empowerment and resources. Motivating the faculty to pursue scholarly projects includes hiring faculty who desire involvement in research, as well as promoting research among novices. On the one hand, chair-endorsed expectations of faculty are important. On the other hand, rewards must also exist, including such things as promotion and tenure, research awards, travel linked to presentation of results, and departmental acknowledgment. Building departmental capacity includes capacity at the departmental level as well as at the individual level. Departmental capacity rests upon an administrative structure for research (e.g. a research division), and includes activities (faculty development, sharing research ideas, publication-development projects, evaluation of research progress, research conferences), research laboratories (clinics, practice-based research networks), and both human (research assistants, scientific writer, biostatistician, epidemiologist), and non-human (pilot funds, computers, software) resources. Individual capacity rests on research-dedicated time, research skill development (fellowship training, faculty development, conferences, skills manuals), and critique (mentorship, research reviews, publication reviews). Opportunities for short-term wins are essential through such activities as promoting rapid publication and recognition awards. Gains must be consolidated and integrated into the activities of the department, anchoring them to the culture (Harris *et al*, 2003).

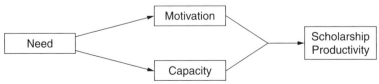

Figure 12.1 From Need to Scholarship.

Rothman and Badyrka (1991) outlined an approach for building entry-level research when no departmental research expertise exists. This interdisciplinary, collaborative, and developmental process relies upon the department's ability to use external researchers to build its own scholarship program. However, the process still requires a stable core of faculty, a willingness to collaborate, and basic resources, such as faculty support, faculty development expertise, seed funds, and teaching flexibility. Initially, departmental faculty form linkages with external researchers through collaborative teaching experiences. Thus, faculty in primary care and psychiatry may co-teach a seminar on depression among primary care patients. Second, when faculty members with similar research interests are identified, these individuals are encouraged to make external presentations and participate in professional meetings. Finally, faculty members are stratified based upon their research expertise, and encouraged to pursue different research paths based upon this level of expertise (Rothman and Badyrka, 1991). Although different research development options are created, research development is concentrated on those faculty members with the greatest interest in research. The research director needs to promote a research paradigm within the department, while trying to increase the level of understanding about primary care research in the chair and dean.

Once research activity has begun within the department, it must be continuously reinforced. Early attention to productivity (e.g. publications) and mentoring relationships is important. Use whatever reinforcing factors are found. Promotion (but not tenure) is a powerful reinforcement to scholarship (Collins, 1993). A total quality management (TQM) approach to fostering research can also be taken (*see* Table 12.1). "Mission" is reflected in the identification of a research focus, the outcomes of which may be the establishment of a collegial environment, the development of mentorship, the recruitment of committed faculty, and the production of relevant research. A "systematic approach" suggests that variation in productivity is minimized, which leads to assessment of strengths and weaknesses, assessment of usefulness, and feedback focused on promoting quality. The "human resources" element means that training and support are essential. This results in prioritization of resource use, and maximizes the number of faculty members involved in research. "Long-term thinking" suggests that a research agenda is valuable, leading to assessment of group needs and appropriate use of resources. Finally, "commitment" mandates institutional and faculty support, resulting in a system supportive of investigation.

Entrepreneurial and Sustainable Research Programs

Perhaps more difficult than establishing a research program is its maintenance. While entrepreneurial programs have cadres of experienced researchers capable of gearing their research to the whims of the National Institutes of Health (NIH), sustainable programs have a specific research focus or agenda, and become recognized for it. Entrepreneurial programs rely upon the diversity of skill sets within its investigators to be able to respond successfully to new directions in funding. Sustainable programs rely upon a wealth of experienced investigators in a single research area with in-depth skills and a track record of successful collaboration.

Table 12.1 TQM Approach to Scholarship Development (Adapted from Paterson *et al*, 1993)

TQM Element	Research Productivity	Outcomes
Mission	Research focus	Relevant research Faculty recruitment Mentoring Collegial environment
Systematic approach	Decrease productivity variation	Identify strengths/weaknesses Assess usefulness Feedback on quality
Human resources	Training and support	Prioritization Increase numbers of researchers
Long-term thinking	Research agenda	Use of resources Needs of group
Commitment	Institutional support Faculty investment	System support

But, once established, keeping the enthusiasm for research and its expansion presents its own challenges. Many programs have established research only to fail to move to the sustainable stage. When providing departmental consultations, the Department of Family and Community Medicine at the University of Missouri evaluates a department's research activities, accomplishments, infrastructure, and organizational environment, so that they can determine the department's strengths, weaknesses, opportunities, and threats relevant to its research program. This information is then used to create an individual development plan for each department.

Collins (1993) suggests that the key to long-term growth is a focus on activities that produce cumulative advantage. First, instead of concentrating on activities that have only short-term effects (e.g. attainment of a prestigious degree or mentor), the research director and investigators need to focus on long-term issues. Flexibility of time and work allow researchers to take advantage of opportunities; research needs to be integrated into teaching responsibilities. Recruitment of researchers who do not need development streamlines the process. Formation of collaborative teams enhances skills and productivity. External funding permits the accumulation of resources. In addition, the research director and individual investigators need to periodically reflect on whether they are accumulating advantages or merely providing service. Ultimately, as these advantages are accumulated, growth becomes multiplicative as in the development of research centers.

The Course of Development

The development of a viable, productive research program does not happen quickly; it requires diligence and patience . . . and a minimum of five years of commitment. But it is possible. DeHaven *et al* (1994) reported on moving a department from no research activity to the acquisition of four research grants, totaling $36,000 in three years and two publications in four years. In San Antonio, we built an active program from one producing a low level of activity, primarily dependent upon collaboration with faculty in other departments. Although the greatest growth occurred over the first three years, there were modest increases after five years (*see* Table 12.2). Figure 12.2 shows the progress in scholarly activity development during the developmental phase. Scholarly activity and presentations surged within the first three years. However, the most prestigious presentations required five years. Publications and grants showed steady progress over the first five years and continued to increase even after five years. As the developmental phase ended and maintenance began (*see* Figure 12.3), the proportion of new or dropped studies as well as those in design phase dropped, while collaborative studies rose. These figures are in general agreement with those of Fairweather (2002) who found that during 1992–93, health sciences faculty averaged 5.1 publications and 5.4 presentations per individual. The message is that development of a research program is a long-term process requiring long-term commitment and diligence; chairs must realize that quick-fix approaches will not work.

Table 12.2 Development of Research Activity in San Antonio

Outcome	Baseline	Development		
		3 Years	*5 Years*	*13 Years*
Scholarly Activity				
Research				
studies	9	91	112	139
collaborative (%)	20	53	67	71
completed (%)	0	45	37	68
faculty involved (%)	28	95	100	81
Non-Research Projects	7	71	74	97
National Presentations				
Total Presentations	2	49	60	75
research papers	0	12	24	19
plenary talks	0	1	5	10
Faculty Presenting (%)	11	49	62	77
Grants				
Grants Submitted	0	12	23	30
Faculty Involved	0	9	12	17
Publications				
Total Publications	9	16	43	93
research papers	2	7	24	37
major articles	9	12	32	58
Faculty Publishing (%)	17	32	52	77

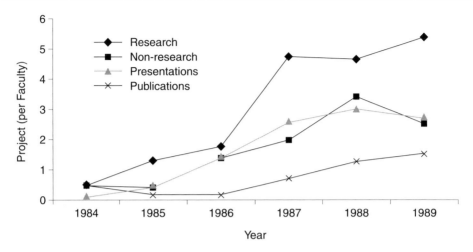

Figure 12.2 Development of Scholarly Activity in San Antonio.

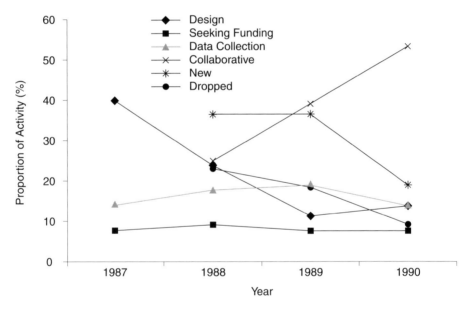

Figure 12.3 Research Activity During the Development Phase.

Synthesis

Developing research in a department *de novo* depends upon both motivation and capacity. Although it is possible to develop research from within, the use of external collaborative relationships may facilitate research development. Thus, novice researchers who co-teach with experienced researchers in other departments may begin to collaborate on research projects, resulting in their own research development. The risk in relying upon external researchers to develop departmental investigators is that these developing researchers may lose their departmental orientation, feeling more attached to the other department.

Once research is established, simply doing "more of the same" will not move the research program to the next level; rather, a specific plan must be developed and implemented. But whatever the goal of research development within the department or residency may be, it represents a long-term commitment and cannot be accomplished overnight. The leadership must acknowledge this commitment up front. Finally, there is no one correct strategy or plan; each department and environment is unique and is going to dictate a unique plan for research development and support (Bland *et al*, 2005).

## Chapter 13

Elements of a Departmental Development Plan

> *Vignette*
>
> K.N. realized that, when initiating a research program where none had existed, she would need to use a variety of strategies and balance activities that would promote research among individual faculty members with activities that would promote research at the departmental level. In addition, if she used faculty time for group meetings, there would be less time available for mentorship and writing manuscripts. So she began by focusing on the building of research culture, using group activities such as mock study sections to build group identity as well as develop individual skills. The emphasis was on the value of group critique to improve the quality of individual projects.

Numerous activities, resources, and policies have been advocated to promote scholarly activity in departments of primary care (*see* Box 13.1). Hollenberg (1992) emphasized the need for personnel (research assistants, secretarial staff, fellows and students, editorial assistant, basic science collaborators), resources (computers, clinical database, space), and funding (pilot funds, travel funds for conferences, external support) to encourage research. But he felt that the importance of protected time and clinical laboratories was over-rated. Instead, he felt that research management skills needed more emphasis, and suggested that research retreats and conferences, critique of presentations and grant proposals, patience and encouragement as well as making people accountable for goals were important to the development of research. In 1980, many departments and residencies reported major impediments to research. More than half of programs reported that faculty time (78%) and funding for time (61%) were impediments; 58% of programs reported that faculty had less than 10% time available for research. In addition, almost half of the programs indicated that lack of research skills in faculty, research role models, and support for staff and supplies were impediments (Parkerson *et al*, 1982).

Box 13.1 Activities, Resources, Policies, and Personnel Intended to Promote Departmental Scholarly Activity

Activities
- Skill development seminars/workshops
- Research forum
- Critical review
- Research conferences
- Writing group
- Mentorship program
- Research awards
- Resident research

Resources
- Computer equipment
- Audiovisual support
- Pilot funds
- Travel funds
- Research laboratories
- Research manual
- Research time
- Sabbatical
- Fellowship

Policies
- Research expectations
- Publication expectations
- Funding expectations
- Research goals
- Research agenda
- Research division
- Incentive program

Personnel
- Research assistants
- Editor
- Epidemiologist
- Biostatistician
- Research committee
- Promotion and tenure committee
- Visiting professorship
- Collaborators

Although the situation in primary care has presumably improved in terms of its support for research, significant impediments continue in many departments and residencies. As of 1997, 39% of community-based and 73% of university-based programs offered protected time to faculty. But time is not enough; many primary care faculty attended medical schools and residencies in which primary care research was not valued. Thus, to overcome inherent impediments to research, rewards must be offered. For example, programs reward research publications

(74–95%), non-research publications (64–93%), and preparation of teaching materials (50–90%) with promotion. Similarly, programs reward national (93–100%) and regional/state (88–96%) presentations through travel time and reimbursement. Rarely is salary or financial bonus used as a research reward (Oeffinger *et al*, 1997).

But support for research must be viewed in a larger context. Because productivity has been linked to variety in career responsibilities, support for research should be viewed as support for career variety. Such variety is supported through opportunities for professional development (supported via travel and funding for development) and through personnel policies. Such policies can support variety via rewards, performance evaluation, workload distribution, and opportunities for leave (Baldwin, 1983).

Although much has been written about factors that promote or impede research development, many such factors have only empiric support for their validity. What evidence is there to support the impact of suggested interventions in developing research within a department?

Evidence-based Interventions

Scholarly Activity

Empirically, we might expect that scholarly activity (research and non-research) would depend upon a variety of factors from personnel (i.e. research faculty, collaborators, mentors, fellows, support staff, epidemiologist) and computer equipment, to research laboratories and agendas. However, there is little research to support this. But there is longitudinal time series data suggesting that a variety of departmental events preceded significant changes in departmental activity. Here in San Antonio, the implementation of a monthly research methods seminar series, and the annual research methods conference (Primary Care Research Methods and Statistics Conference) was associated with increases in departmental research activity. Similarly, monthly opportunities to present research ideas to other researchers for critique were also linked to increases in research activity. In addition, administrative policies had an impact. While formalizing expectations for research by all faculty preceded an increase in departmental research, establishment of departmental research goals was linked to increases in both research and non-research activity (Katerndahl, 1996). Thus, although some support exists for what we might expect empirically, other factors may also impact the development of scholarship.

Presentations

Presentations at national conferences may depend upon the availability of travel funds and audiovisual support as well as personnel (i.e. research faculty, collaborators, mentors, fellows). There is evidence that a faculty development program of seminars and mentorship (Morzinski and Simpson, 2003), or faculty evaluation focused on feedback and pay decisions (Bland *et al*, 2002) can increase departmental presentations. In San Antonio, the availability of travel funds was linked to increased departmental presentations. As might be expected, when we hosted the North American Primary Care Research Group (NAPCRG) meeting, there was a significant rise in submissions for presentation (Katerndahl, 1996).

Publications

Empirically, the production of manuscripts (and ultimately publications) may depend upon departmental scholarly activity and presentations, as well as faculty time and the availability of a scientific editor. Although programs using faculty development seminars or workshops to increase publications have produced mixed results (Holloway *et al*, 1988; Hekelman *et al*, 1995a; Morzinski and Simpson, 2003), faculty evaluation focused on feedback, and pay decisions increased publications (Bland *et al*, 2002). In addition, the use of mentors (Mills *et al*, 1995; Morzinski and Simpson, 2003), and departmental writing groups (Katerndahl, 1996; Grzybowski *et al*, 2003) has been associated with increases in manuscript submissions and publications. In San Antonio, administrative policy that formally stated expectations of faculty publication was linked to increases in departmental publications (Katerndahl, 1996). Such global findings may explain the association between departmental publications and departmental funding through the receipt of Academic Administrative Units (Health Resources and Services Administration (HRSA)) grants (Wagner *et al*, 1994).

Grants

External research funding, especially from federal sources, may depend upon several factors. In addition to the availability of research laboratories and pilot funds, successful grantsmanship may depend upon research and grant-writing skills, as well as departmental reputation. While such research and grant-writing skills should depend upon collaborators, mentors, faculty development, and the availability of epidemiologists and scientific editors, departmental reputation will depend upon global factors such as the departmental research faculty, their presentation and publication records, the departmental research agenda, awards received, and perhaps access to a practice-based research network. However, little research on predictors of departmental funding has been done. Although research activity, mentors (Mills *et al*, 1995), and faculty feedback have been linked to increased funding (Baldwin *et al*, 1994; Bland *et al*, 2002), such critical review may increase funding at the expense of publications (Baldwin *et al*, 1994).

Summary

Thus, certain patterns across scholarly outcomes are seen. Faculty development, mentorship and critique, and administrative interventions have been successful in promoting departmental scholarly productivity. This may explain why such global events as establishment of a division of research, and protected group time for collaboration were linked to increases in non-research scholarship as well as publications and presentations in San Antonio. In addition, research conferences such as annual departmental conferences or hosting a NAPCRG meeting may increase communications (publications and presentations), yet providing faculty with a research manual and research assistant availability have not been linked to any scholarly outcomes (Katerndahl, 1996). The availability of resources may be over-rated in the quest to promote scholarship when compared with faculty development and administrative support.

Beyond Simple Interventions

Organizational Structure

In addition to the associations between research-related administrative factors (e.g. the creation of a division of research) and scholarly activity, other administrative factors may impact scholarship. For example, Kohlenberg (1992) found that, while such administrative factors were not correlated with nursing publications or editing activity, administrative structure and procedural specifications were inversely correlated with both research and total scholarly activity, and "impersonality" of administration was inversely related to total scholarship. The inverse relationship between non-research administration and scholarship was suggested by Katerndahl (1996). The institution of a family medicine clerkship for students was associated with a decline in scholarly activity and communications. Thus, scholarship can be affected by other departmental administrative events; research is part of the departmental whole.

Personnel

Although both empirical and experimental work supports the importance of personnel in scholarly activity, the role of research-related personnel in the process of building research capacity is not always clear-cut. As mentioned above, the availability of research assistants was not associated with increased scholarship (Katerndahl, 1996). Similarly, although the presence of a research fellowship within a department would be expected to promote departmental scholarship, it comes at a price. Curtis *et al* (1998) estimated that National Research Service Award (NRSA) primary care research fellowships cost their departments almost $15,000 to run. This represents a considerable investment during times of limited financing. Along similar lines, the endowment of a research chair is not necessarily a boon to research within a department. When social scientists rated the priorities for endowed research chairs, "conducting research" was not rated as its primary purpose; the purpose of the endowed research chair was seen to be primarily as an administrative tool or role model, and the foremost day-to-day activity of this chair was seen to be in teaching (McNeely *et al*, 1987). Thus, the benefits to scholarship of research-related personnel and their programs are not always clear.

Faculty Career Advancement

Finally, as with any measure of scholarship, simple interventions may not produce improvement; multiple interventions may be necessary. To promote faculty success in promotion and tenure, departmental programs need to not only encourage faculty grants and communications, but university service and involvement in national organizations as well. Faculty awards may also be important. Although a program of departmental awards is helpful, departments may need to actively seek national awards for its faculty through programs to encourage scholarly communications, mentorship, a research agenda, and sabbaticals. Although little research has focused on such activities, a multilevel program for career advancement may be necessary.

Such a program was implemented to correct gender bias in career advancement. The program included obvious interventions such as faculty education, faculty development, evaluation, mentorship, and rewards, but also included interventions for leaders (leader support, implementation task force, external consultant) and activities to decrease isolation of women faculty members (meetings, retreats, committee involvement). After three years, improvements in ratings were found in the areas of timely promotions, gender bias, access to career information, sense of isolation, and salary equity. Women faculty members rated their mentors and departmental support more highly after the three years, their expectations for promotion and plans to stay in academia improved, and more had received promotion to associate professor (Fried *et al*, 1996). Such multilevel programs in career development do work.

Synthesis

Although this chapter may suggest, and what little research exists may support, the idea that simple interventions may promote scholarship within departments, such simple interventions have a low likelihood of success. As complex systems, departments consist of varied faculty members, involved in varied activities and hence will respond differently to different interventions. Thus, a program of multiple interventions carries the greatest likelihood of success (*see* Section IV). Departmental activities and events must be viewed as interventions, experiments with measured outcomes which may or may not contribute to the research endeavor, and which can be discarded if not productive.

## Chapter 14

Departmental Resources: Mentors, Money and Models

Vignette

She was ready to give up! Clearly, the junior investigators in the department needed mentorship and, clearly, she alone couldn't provide it all. But all of her efforts to get junior faculty to identify a mentor had failed. It was time for drastic action . . . a structured mentorship program! So K.N. identified a group of senior faculty with the qualities desired in mentors and elicited their participation. Then she assigned mentor–protégé pairs and found a time slot in which they could regularly meet . . . and crossed her fingers.

Departmental Mentorship

As mentioned in Section II, there are many benefits of mentorship, and having a mentor is a predictor of academic success. Yet, there is less mentorship in clinical disciplines than in those of the basic sciences. This is especially true of primary care. Not only has the changing structure of practice impeded mentorship, but the high turnover rate makes it difficult to form long-term relationships. The "good old boy" networks that support ongoing mentoring relations do not exist anymore. In addition, there is a strong sense of independence and self-reliance that pressures young investigators to try to do it on their own. Finally, clinical academicians simply have more stress and less time available than their basic science counterparts. These factors are even truer in primary care. Add in the fact that family medicine is only 30 years old, and grew out of a clinical rather than research tradition, and it becomes obvious that primary care researchers have few mentorship opportunities; there are very few seasoned, successful investigators capable of serving as mentors. However, in light of the burning need for and benefits of mentorship, we must find a way to provide this nurturance to less experienced investigators.

Mentoring

Junior faculty need mentoring. Not only does mentoring predict academic success, but junior faculty need to adopt academic values, establish productive networks of colleagues, and manage their careers (Virginia Commonwealth University, 1997). However, for a mentoring relationship to be productive, a protégé must display certain characteristics. Attitudinally, the protégé must be eager to learn from the mentor, serious about the relationship, flexible and understanding about the availability of the mentor's time, and accepting of criticism. In addition, the protégé needs to be prompt for meetings and proactive about the relationship, willing to seek mentors, able to define his/her needs for a mentor, and able to identify experts in his/her field (Rogers *et al*, 1990; Stange and Hekelman, 1990; Virginia Commonwealth University, 1997).

But the benefits of a mentoring relationship are not one-way; mentors benefit as well. In addition to the personal sense of satisfaction inherent in helping a junior faculty member to succeed, mentoring enables mentors to improve their own managerial skills and provides the opportunity for joint projects. On a higher plane, mentorship provides the opportunity to extend the mentor's work, and to bridge to future generations. On a practical note, research suggests that junior faculty are more likely to include others as co-authors if they have been good collaborators in the past or have some administrative power (Mainous *et al*, 2002), suggesting that protégés will be predisposed to include you as a co-author if your mentoring relationship is a good one. Shapiro *et al* (1994) found that senior faculty motivations to serve as mentors tend to be oriented to benefits for the institution or the relationship. While senior faculty, non-tenured faculty, and faculty with previous mentorship experience are all likely to intend to serve as mentors, they are also likely to see the potential drawbacks as well (Ragins and Cotton, 1993).

The characteristics of a good mentor are easy to list. In addition to being experienced, networked, and academically successful, a good mentor should be empathetic and challenging, with a sense of vision (Perkoff, 1992). Typically, a good mentor–protégé relationship will share common professional interests, common personal interests, and mutual respect.

The mentor can serve in several capacities: teaching the protégé, supporting the protégé, sponsoring the protégé, or intervening on the protégé's behalf. Ultimately, the mentor is there to facilitate the protégé's learning, not provide solutions. However, mentors' roles tend to fall into one of four categories. Tenured mentors tend to serve as friends, while mentors in graduate schools tend to serve as intellectual guides. Female mentors often serve as sources of information or career guides (Sands *et al*, 1991). Thus, it is common and appropriate to have more than one mentor, or a series of mentors as the protégé's needs change (Rogers *et al*, 1990).

The mentorship process should follow a somewhat standard formula. Mentors need to encourage an open, trusting relationship, offer time and information, and encourage the protégé to outgrow the need for a mentor. Mentors should be positive and supportive, demonstrate confidence in protégés, facilitate networking, admit ignorance, and provide frequent honest feedback. This is supported by the research of Palepu *et al* (1998) who found that protégés identified mentors' commitment to protégés' careers (88%), mentors' ability to motivate (66%), mentors' research skills (49%), and mentors' contacts and networking (43%) as factors contributing to the effectiveness of the mentorship. Protégés need to identify their goals, meet regularly with the mentor, listen to advice without being overly sensitive to criticism, and keep the relationship professional without betraying confidences. Specifically, mentors should establish regular meetings, identify protégés' expectations and verbalize their own, discuss the institution's promotion and tenure policies, and allow protégés to collaborate with them on projects (Virginia Commonwealth University, 1997). Senior faculty use socialization and the relationship to meet the mentorship goals (Shapiro *et al*, 1994). Thus, Cohen (1995) suggests that while the mentor's modeling serves to motivate, and the protégé's goals provide the initiative, an emphasis on the relationship establishes trust. A facilitative focus opens alternatives while a well-timed confrontative focus provides challenge. The influence that the mentorship experience has on success depends upon the trust and timing of confrontations. Hence, early in the process, the emphasis should be on the relationship to build trust. Later, the emphasis is on advice, and then facilitation and confrontation. Finally, the mentor must always be moving the protégé towards a transition to independence.

Bower *et al* (1998) suggest that the results of mentorship are based on the balance between support and challenge. A lack of support and challenge leads to stasis, while support without challenge provides only confirmation, and challenge without support leads to a sense of failure. Only a balance of support with challenge leads to growth driven by the vision that the mentor–protégé pair brings to the relationship. Consequently, the protégés need to continually evaluate their mentorship in terms of regularity of meetings, encouragement and feedback received, advocacy by the mentor to departmental leadership, involvement in mentors' projects, facilitation of protégés' involvement in national organizations, collaborations, and networks, and challenge to develop research ideas, and submit grants and manuscripts (Virginia Commonwealth University, 1997). Beware of situations in which mentors want protégés to further their agenda or serve as research assistants without appropriate credit, promote unethical behavior, expect authorship on protégés' manuscripts without contributing, or provide inappropriate praise or criticism. Any of these signs suggest that the relationship needs to end. Finally, mentors should always be in the process of moving protégés toward becoming independent researchers; failing to make this transition will ultimately be detrimental to protégés.

Mentorship Programs

When establishing a departmental mentorship program, you must start with an environment that encourages collaboration. This can be more difficult than it sounds because there are often inherent barriers within departments and institutions. Such barriers include jealousy, geographic separation, and financial reasons, as well as differences in promotion criteria and grant support (Mukamal *et al*, 2002). However, as Table 14.1 shows, there are strategies for promoting collaboration within departments and institutions. As research director, you need to encourage supportive faculty interaction via social activities, faculty development, promotion of interaction and cross-fertilization, and clinical peer review. The departmental chair can further support collaboration through inclusive governance, acknowledging the value of integration, faculty evaluation, provision of support staff, and development of centers of excellence, and financial measures such as rewarding collaboration, providing incentives, and compensating equitably. Finally, medical schools can encourage interdisciplinary collaboration via comparable promotional criteria, educator–researcher pairings, and incentives (Mukamal *et al*, 2002). When initiating a mentorship program, the provision of a conducive environment is again essential. Thus, the research

Table 14.1 Strategies That Encourage Collaboration (Adapted from Mukamal *et al*, 2002)

Faculty	*Leaders*	*Medical School*
Promote each other	Acknowledge the value of integration	Identical academic ranks
Faculty development	Compensate equitably	Pair educators and researchers
Mentorship program	Appropriate financial incentives	Publication as an incentive
Encourage cross-fertilization	Inclusive governance	
Clinical peer review	Reward collaborative leaders	
Social activities	Centers of excellence	
	Facilitate evaluation of support staff	

director and chair should encourage an open environment, facilitate interactions between junior and senior faculty, explicitly plan career paths, and provide opportunities for faculty to network with faculty outside of the department (Stange and Hekelman, 1990). Once the department is prepared, recruitment of mentors and protégés can begin, keeping in mind the characteristics of good mentors, and the requirements of the mentor–protégé relationship as presented above. Protégés are then oriented to the program, receive workshop training concerning mentorship, and select their mentors. Protégés are prompted to contact their chosen mentor, mentor–protégé pairs are provided with recommendations for mentorship activities, and the research director monitors progress, prepared to make revisions as necessary (Morzinski *et al*, 1994).

Although ideally mentor–protégé pairings should form spontaneously, as we found in San Antonio, sometimes encouragement is not enough and a formal mentorship program needs to be established, which may even include assignment of mentors to protégés. Mentorship programs should include goals and priorities, standards for mentors and their roles, criteria for selecting and matching protégés, policies and procedures for implementation, training and rewards for mentors, tools for evaluation, and resources for implementation (Morahan, 2001). Obviously, both mentors and protégés, as well as the chair, must ''buy into'' the process for it to succeed. Sufficient time must be available for mentors and protégés to meet frequently, and departments must recognize the need to invest in the development of their junior faculty. In a program that assigns mentors and protégés, there must be enough supervision for evaluation of relationships, and flexibility to change assignments if they are not productive (Virginia Commonwealth University, 1997).

Sometimes, internal mentorship programs do not work, either because senior internal faculty will not serve as mentors, or because there are insufficient numbers of senior faculty suitable as mentors. In this case, external mentors are needed. External mentors should be chosen based on a match in content area, and can be drawn from any discipline. If appropriate mentors cannot be found at the protégé's institution, it may be necessary to seek mentors from other institutions. In this case, mentors and protégés commit to a one-year participation with periodic meetings at the mentor's institution or at professional meetings. Financial support for such an external mentorship program is critical. Not only are funds needed for travel for the protégé, but the availability of funds enables mentors to receive an honorarium, for expert consultation and reviews. In addition, frequent mentor–protégé interaction via email and telephone is encouraged. However, mentors must be carefully selected based upon review of the mentor's curriculum vitae (CV), discussion with the mentor, and appropriateness of the matching. The research director, chair, or dean must be responsible for selection of mentors. As difficult as such an external mentorship program may seem, such a program has demonstrated success over a 2.5-year period in terms of publications, presentations, and funded grant proposals (Mundt, 2001).

Whatever system is used, a continuous pipeline of productive researchers cannot be established within a department without a viable mentorship program. Although the research director can serve as mentor for a few junior faculty, once a core of active researchers is established, additional mentors will be needed and a mentorship program, whether formal or informal, will be a necessity.

Resource Management

One of the key responsibilities of the research director is the securing and management of resources in support of research. Resource management is particularly critical in times of resource scarcity, such as now. In fact, among professionals involved in paradigm development of their disciplines, attitudes about the value of research and perceived criticality of resources were particularly strong (McKinley *et al*, 1986). Thus, leaders in the process of fostering development of a discipline recognize the need for resource management if the discipline is to continue to mature. This is no less true for primary care or a department committed to advancement.

Funding Support

Financial support is always important to the success of any research venture. Although it is true that some research can be achieved without strong financial support, most of the truly important studies will need enough funding for the inclusion of sufficient numbers of subjects for sufficiently long periods of time to produce meaningful and convincing results. Aside from the number of departmental faculty, departmental support via Academic Administrative Units (AAU) grants from the Health Resources and Services Administration (HRSA) was a strong predictor of departmental publications (Wagner *et al*, 1994). But the reality is that primary care research is poorly funded. In 1980, 51 family medicine programs received a total of $3.5 million for research, 75% of which came from governmental sources (Parkerson *et al*, 1982). But this poor level of funding support from federal agencies has not improved much, judging by the lack of support for family medicine research in the recent budgets of the Agency for Healthcare Research and Quality (AHRQ), and the National Institutes of Health (NIH) (Campos-Outcalt and Senf, 1999). Thus, primary care departments must intentionally seek to develop a cadre of researchers with the capability of securing federal funding, and must look for creative alternative sources of research support.

Financial support for departmental research is critical. These funds pay for pilot studies, maintenance and operations (M&O), equipment such as computers and software, and travel to national meetings. These are the basics. All departments active in research have these infrastructure expenses. Without financial support for these functions, research cannot flourish. Where these funds come from is another matter.

Active mature research programs generate these funds through their federal grants either as core funds of a center grant or as pieces of multiple R01s. But few primary care departments can secure such funding this way. Traditionally, family medicine departments have used HRSA's AAU grants for this purpose. In addition, the other Title VII grants can be used to supplement the AAU grants if their proposed focus relates to research. Another potential source of infrastructure support is contracts. Contracts may be particularly useful when the subject of the contract deals with a research focus of the department, thus reinforcing current research. However, contracts take time, and may therefore be counterproductive if they do not relate to the interests of the department. Pharmaceutical companies may also provide some limited support. For example, a department could use an unrestricted educational grant for faculty develop-ment.

Finally, if possible, indirect funds can be used to support infrastructure; in fact, this is their intent. Indirect funds attached to a research grant are supposed to support the infrastructure that underpins all research. Thus, departments should receive these funds whenever they secure grants. However, many institutions appropriate these funds for institutional support. If they do return them to the department, chairs may use them for general infrastructure needs and not return them for research infrastructure. Thus, if possible, the research director should lobby for the return of indirect funds to the research division as ongoing support for the research endeavor.

Human Resources

Faculty who value research perceive staff support as being more critical than do faculty who do not value research (McKinley *et al*, 1986). Not only are secretaries needed to type manuscripts and grants, arrange travel, and keep records, but a variety of other support personnel are also essential. Trained, skilled, experienced research assistants are the backbone of the research enterprise. Research assis-tants can make or break a research study.

In a mature research division, an ongoing stream of grants supports well-trained research assistants. But in a fledgling research effort, support for research assistants may be hard to come by. Thus, research directors must be open to other sources of basic research personnel. Work-study programs may permit data entry-level personnel to be hired cheaply from high schools and colleges. Medical students can also be used as research assistants. Finally, graduate students from local graduate schools may serve as research assistants, using the studies as a source for their theses and dissertations. Unfortunately, these solutions are only short-term remedies, and require time investment from investigators in order to train these assistants.

Research divisions also need personnel with advanced skill sets. Active research units depend heavily upon their computer systems for data management, communication, and analysis. Therefore, computer support personnel are essen-tial to research divisions to ensure that computers stay online. In addition, scientific editors play a role in the production and refinement of manuscripts and grants. Such editors can also train secretaries to streamline the process of manuscript production. Finally, although few departments have them and funding agencies will not pay for them, grant writers may be a valuable addition to the staff. These specialists can provide the non-scientific portion of the first draft of the grant, review the ongoing stream of funding opportunities available, and polish the final version of the grant proposal to maximize its chances of funding.

But research endeavors also need access to specialized research skills. There-fore, research units must have access to biostatisticians and epidemiologists. Such skill sets are often essential in the planning of fundable projects, and may be required parts of a successful research team. If the department cannot hire such individuals, then access to them must be arranged within the institution.

External Support

Often the resources you need cannot be found within your department, and the funds to secure them cannot be obtained. In that case, you must look outside for resources. As research director, it is important for you to establish relationships throughout your institution and the discipline.

Other departments, especially older departments with a strong tradition of research, may be a source of resources. Although such resources may include funding for pilot work, generally such external resources are human resources – collaborators and mentors, research assistants, and editors. Although it may be possible to collaborate with other departments of primary care at other institutions, generally such external collaborations will involve non-primary care departments within your institution. As long as responsibilities are clearly delineated up front, such collaborations can be very productive and mutually beneficial.

Within your institution, other opportunities for resources may exist. In addition to institutional grants programs, all academic institutions have institutional review boards (IRBs) to ensure the safety of research subjects, and offices of grants management (OGMs) to manage grant funds secured by institutional faculty. Lesson number one in dealing with these bodies is that you need them more than they need you, so a confrontational approach in dealing with them is counterproductive; studies cannot begin until approved by the IRB, and grant proposals cannot be submitted until approved by the OGM. Play nice! The second lesson is that they may be able to help you as research director. Not only may both bodies offer informal (or even formal) instruction in protection of human subjects and grant preparation, but they can help investigators on an individual basis. Hence, IRB leadership can often suggest methodological ways to obtain sensitive data while minimizing risk to subjects. OGM staff can help investigators locate potential funding sources for particular projects. In addition, if your institution has offices of computing and educational resources, these can also be sources of support. Offices of computing resources typically provide instruction in computer software packages and establishment of email lists as well as statistical support. Similarly, offices of educational resources usually provide faculty development activities that may include research, writing, and grantmanship skill development. Thus, your institution may be able to provide you with some of the human resources and instruction that your department needs.

Finally, the discipline of family medicine has recently embraced the need for research as never before. Consequently, organizations within the discipline may be able to help. The American Academy of Family Physicians (AAFP) recently ended its cycle of Advanced Research Training grants but may offer them again. Both the Society of Teachers of Family Medicine (STFM) and the North American Primary Care Research Group (NAPCRG) offer skill development in research and statistics. In addition, NAPCRG's Grant Generating Project has proven remarkably successful at stimulating grant submissions and funding among established researchers. Attendance at the Primary Care Research Methods and Statistics Conference is associated with increased publications and grant submissions (Katerndahl, 2000a). Finally, the AAFP Foundation and many of its state foundations offer small research grants to support pilot projects. Thus, the discipline itself may be able to provide instructional and funding support to your investigators.

Cultivating Research Laboratories

Ultimately, for clinical research to occur, you must have access to research subjects (patients). Although you may be able to access patients through collaborators or conduct community-based research via door-to-door or telephone methods, the easiest access to patients is through the use of clinical settings within your department. Although generally consisting of resident or faculty primary care patients, departmental clinical populations may also include clinics and practices linked into research networks. The availability of multiple research sites and varied research settings can facilitate scholarly activity, increase departmental reputation (and ultimately funding), and promote the development of research centers.

Residency Clinics

Ambulatory training is at the heart of primary care education. The patient population in residency clinics serves as the study population for much of primary care research. Patients seen by faculty versus residents differ in some clinical and demographic ways. Patients seeing residents have more head, eyes, ears, nose, and throat (HEENT), respiratory, and genitourinary problems, but fewer dermatological problems. In addition, they are more likely to have Medicaid and present for maternity care, but less likely to be older and non-Hispanic white, and have Medicare or private insurance (Scheid *et al*, 1995). However, in general, patients seen in residency practices are similar to private primary care patients in terms of reasons-for-visit, diagnoses, hospitalization rates, and duration-of-visit (Gilchrist *et al*, 1993). Thus, results from residency-based research can be generalizable to practice settings.

But to facilitate the use of residency patients as research subjects, you need to collect standardized information during office visits and maintain the data in comprehensive databases. Hence, the use of electronic medical records with standardized collection of basic information on all patients at all visits facilitates the development of an easily-accessed, high-quality, research database capable of generating valid pilot study results quickly. This database can be further enhanced by regular collection of brief, but high-impact, outcomes information, such as a measure of quality of life. These simple measures can turn a clinical billing database into a research database, capable of answering important primary care research questions. Coincidentally, these same high-impact outcomes data can be extremely useful in quality assurance studies and resident evaluation, thus serving multiple purposes.

FIRMS

The concept of firm systems (FIRMS) seeks to turn a primary care clinic setting into a site for randomized studies. FIRMS are based on certain principles, emphasizing the provision of continuity of care during longitudinal studies. They use the random assignment of both physicians and patients to modules within the clinic to serve as a proxy for randomization within the study design. Then, different interventions can be instituted within different modules and ultimately compared.

For FIRMS to work, the different modules must be geographically isolated to prevent contamination, and the size of the modules must be kept small (maximum of 12 physicians per module). In addition, sample size adjustments must be made in FIRMS studies because patients are randomized as groups, necessitating larger numbers of subjects (Cebul, 1991). The beauty of the FIRMS system is the ability to conduct randomized trials using a variety of atypical interventions, such as behavioral and administrative interventions. The downside is that FIRMS must be maintained at an expense of time and effort while permitting patients to "opt out" of random assignment if they choose a particular physician.

Networks

Practice-Based Research Networks

The practice-based research network (PBRN) is a unique research tool developed by family medicine, but now includes networks in internal medicine, pediatrics (Beasley, 1993), and psychiatry (Zarin *et al*, 1997). As of 1993, there were 26 primary care research networks (Beasley, 1993). In fact, many state academies of family practice run their own research networks. The obvious benefits of PBRNs include their representativeness of the primary care and US populations (Green *et al*, 1984), as well as their ability to study practice variation. Recently, federal sources of grant support have shown an interest in PBRNs as a source of research subjects.

PBRNs require ongoing support to grow and maintain their participating physicians. With strong volunteer support, a PBRN can probably be launched with $50 000 per year for three years as seed money (Green and Lutz, 1990). Key features needed to develop and maintain a successful network include regular meetings and communication, a lack of intrusiveness of studies into practices, and involvement of participating physicians in development of research questions and design.

Physicians join a research network for a variety of reasons. A desire to contribute to developing new knowledge and to be part of a group engaged in research is the most frequently cited reason. However, some physicians join in order to discuss research ideas, for the possibility of seeing findings implemented into practice, or to obtain information about how others practice (Osborn and Pettiti, 1988; Green *et al*, 1991). Based largely upon the experience of the Ambulatory Sentinel Practice Network (ASPN), about 10% of practices will leave a PBRN each year (although 13% rejoin later). The most common reasons for withdrawing from a PBRN are a change in the practice, the burden associated with PBRN involvement, and lack of support from colleagues and staff. Fortunately, 70% of ASPN practices were still involved eight years after joining (Green *et al*, 1991).

Thus, one method for expanding the number and diversity of research sites available is to develop a PBRN. Although requiring some financial and considerable time investment, its benefits are well accepted and have finally drawn the attention of funding agencies.

Residency Networks

An alternative to development of a PBRN is the residency-based research network. A residency-based research network links several residency programs together into a research network. This is a natural development for large departments with several affiliated residency programs. Not only does the department benefit through the addition of residency research sites, but affiliated programs benefit in their accreditation by having faculty involved in research.

Although concerns about the generalizability of research results from residency-based studies exist, the residency patient populations are similar to clinical populations within their areas. In addition, several institutional review boards may need to approve studies, causing considerable delay. As with any network-based study, adjustments in sample size calculations must be made. However, the benefits of such residency-based networks include the ability to collect data on many subjects over relatively short time intervals, and the exposure that residents get to the research process. With relatively little investment from component residencies, a residency-based research network can be very productive.

Academic Center Networks

One form of research network that has not been adequately pursued is that of linking academic departments of primary care into a research network. Although the AAFP-funded research centers have involved collaborative efforts among a few departments, this is a long way from the collaborative research network models of the South West Oncology Group (SWOG), for example. This highly productive oncology research network should be a model for such academic research networks. Such networks could bring together highly productive individual primary care researchers with different skills to pursue research areas critical to primary care.

Synthesis

Resources, resources, and resources! Research programs must have resources such as mentors, support, and laboratories. Although mentor–protégé relationships should ideally develop naturally, mentorship is too important to a department's research effort to be left to chance. Thus, a departmental mentorship program may be needed, with mentors who are chosen with care, and relationships that are nurtured and allowed to blossom.

Although the best approach is to secure *all* of the other resources you need from your Chair, guaranteed for at least five years, this is not likely to happen. In this case, you will need to be able to secure funding and human resources to move the research endeavor forward. Often such plans will need to take advantage of resources within your institution and the discipline if you are to be successful.

Finally, research laboratories must be cultivated if a department is to be productive. Routine clinical activity should be conducted with an eye on the potential for future use of clinical records for research. Multiple research sites provide flexibility to pursue a variety of research questions while promoting the reputation (and fundability) of its researchers. Although practice-based research networks have finally "come of age" and are receiving federal recognition, linking residencies and departments into research networks may also be valuable.

## Chapter 15

Evaluating Success

Vignette

After three years, K.N. was disheartened. As she prepared for her annual meeting with the chair, she dreaded what would happen. She knew that her publications had dropped and that her only major funding was her Health Resources and Services Administration (HRSA) grant. But, as she sat down across from the chair, he was elated. Departmental research studies, funding, and publications had quadrupled in the past two years! Even other chairs were acknowledging the change to him. She had forgotten the first rule of being a director of research; it's not about you and your productivity, it's about the productivity of the department.

Evaluation is critical! The development of a research program is, at best, a five-year commitment. In addition, different aspects of the program develop at different rates, so the fact that National Institutes of Health (NIH) funding has not increased after three years is not a sign of failure. Finally, not everyone's definition of "success" is the same. If the research program is evaluated at regular intervals, then progress in different areas can be monitored, demonstrating which areas are progressing and which may need added attention. Also, if the chair's singular definition of "success" is not advancing, you can still show that overall progress is being made. Finally, regular evaluation provides data that can be very useful as justification for training or development grants.

Before measuring success, we need to state traditional assumptions, many of which may not be true. Focusing on publications and citations, the first assumption is that the more the publications the better. Second, there is a direct relationship between the quantity and quality of publications, and between the quality of the publication and the number of its citations. Third, well-known authors attract citations beyond the merit of their current publication. Fourth, publications in English-American journals are cited more frequently. Finally, some subjects are cited more than others (Luukonen, 1990). Whether these assumptions are true is a matter of conjecture, but they often color our interpretation. If these assumptions are wrong, then our assessments may miss the mark; truly important, innovative, and ultimately seminal work may not be recognized.

In addition, it is also important to remember that different institutions may need different scales of success. Wallace (1990) found that the publication rate at research universities varied considerably, and that the presence of a doctoral program had a significant impact on publication rate. Thus, when interpreting specific measures of success, we should probably avoid the temptation to compare our results with those of other institutions, because the frame of reference may be different.

Measures of Success

During our development phase, we began collecting detailed information about the scholarly activity of the department. Faculty members completed an annual scholarly activity survey, describing their scholarship during the previous 12 months (*see* Appendix 1). Although initially done based on the fiscal year, this was changed to the calendar year to facilitate identification of when publications and presentations were made. Although faculty differed in the speed of their response, nagging or interviewing ultimately produced a 100% response rate.

This survey elicited information about each active research and non-research scholarly project, including the name of the project, co-investigators, the current stage at which the project was (from planning to completion), and any presentation and/or manuscript submissions. For each publication, we asked the name of the journal/book and its type (i.e. book chapter, research article, editorial); for each presentation, we asked the name of the conference and its type (i.e. research presentation, plenary talk, poster). For each grant submission, faculty provided the name of the grant, collaborators, type of grant (i.e. research, training), the funding agency, the direct funds requested, and its status (i.e. approved but not funded, pending review). Finally, we asked about review experience for journals, conferences, and study sections.

Analysis of these data involved calculations of indices that were more helpful for assessment (*see* Box 15.1), for example, the proportion of faculty involved in research and non-research, the numbers of projects per faculty, the proportion of research projects involving collaboration, the number of research stages completed since the previous year, the proportion of manuscript submissions accepted for publication, and the proportion of grant submissions funded. Such indices were calculated for the department as a whole in order to assess progress in departmental research development. In addition, they were calculated for each faculty member as part of faculty development, and fed back to the faculty members so that they could assess their individual progress in comparison with the previous year's results and with the anonymous results of other faculty members.

Box 15.1 Indices Calculated from Scholarship Data

Departmental

Research
- Proportion of faculty involved
- Projects per faculty
- Research stages
  - projects at each stage
  - faculty at each stage
- Study progress
  - new studies
  - dropped studies
  - no progress
  - number of stages advanced

- Status of completed projects
  - submissions in preparation
  - presentation/manuscript submissions/acceptances
- Collaboration
  - studies involving internal/external collaboration
  - faculty involved in internal/external collaboration

Non-research
- Proportion of faculty involved
- Projects/faculty
- Status of completed projects
  - submissions in preparation
  - presentation/manuscript submissions/acceptances
- Collaboration
  - studies involving internal/external collaboration
  - faculty involved in internal/external collaboration

Communications
- Publications
  - proportion of faculty publishing
  - publications per faculty
  - acceptance rate
  - proportion of publications in primary care publications
- Presentations
  - proportion of faculty presenting
  - presentations per faculty
  - acceptance rate
  - proportion of presentations at primary care conferences
- Communications per faculty
- Proportion of communications as publications

Grants
- Proportion of submissions to national agencies
- Proportion of submissions to private foundations
- Proportion funded
- Directs per submission
- Directs per funded grant

Reviews
- Proportion of faculty reviewing
- Reviews per faculty

Individual

Research
- Number of projects
- Progress
  - new studies
  - dropped studies
  - total stages advanced
- Collaboration
  - studies involving internal collaboration
  - studies involving external collaboration

Continued

Non-research
- Number of projects

Communications
- Publications
  - submitted
  - accepted
- Presentations
  - number made

Grants
- Submitted
- Funded

Finally, using the Web of Science online, based upon data from the Science Citation Index (SCI) and the Social Science Citation Index (SSCI), we identified the number and sites in which our faculty's publications were cited in the previous year. Such citation information, recognizing that it is limited by the incompleteness of the journals included in the SCI and SSCI, was shared with the faculty and the departmental promotion and tenure committee.

Other authors have also recommended additional measures. These could include membership on research-related committees, graduate student sponsorship, and awards received (Collins, 1993).

Benchmarks Based On Goals

Rating Publications

Not all publications are created equal. Martin and Irvine (1983) suggested that the true worth of a paper was based upon its quality, its importance, and its impact. Quality relates to the rigor of its methods and can only be evaluated by reviewers. One measure of quality would be the speed with which it is accepted for publication. Importance deals with the potential of the paper to influence the advancement of knowledge. Because importance relates to potential, only reviewers can assess importance. Impact, however, deals with whether that potential was realized and can be evaluated, based on where the paper was published and its citations.

Thus, one measure of impact would be based on ratings of journals. In 1982, family physician educators rated the top ten medical journals as shown in Box 15.2. Another approach to rating journals is based upon their citation rates. The SCI and the SSCI publish the Journal Citation Reports annually which list medical journals based upon the frequency with which their articles are cited in other journals (impact factor), and the speed with which their articles are cited in other journals (immediacy factor). Thus, a rating of journals could also be based on their impact and/or immediacy factors (Vieira and Faraino, 1997). Another method for assessing impact is based upon the circulation of the journal in which the publication occurs. Finally, a direct measure of impact is the frequency with which an article is cited in other articles. Hence, simply counting the numbers of publications may not yield the type of information a research director needs for evaluation.

Box 15.2 Top Ten Medical Journals as Rated by Family Physician Educators
(Adapted from Miller, 1982)

1. *Journal of Family Practice*
2. *New England Journal of Medicine*
3. *American Family Physician*
4. *Journal of the American Medical Association*
5. *Annals of Internal Medicine*
6. *Academic Medicine*
7. *Postgraduate Medicine*
8. *Patient Care*
9. *Continuing Education for the Family Physician*
10. *Lancet*

Weighting and Expectations

Raw data concerning scholarly productivity may not address the questions behind the evaluation. Counting manuscript submissions and publications does not tell you the rate of manuscript acceptance for publication. Thus, using the raw data to calculate relevant measures of productivity may yield truly useful figures. One such measure of balance in research progress is the difference between the number of new studies and the number of inactivated studies. Another is the ratio between research and non-research projects. Because a research paper is not equivalent to a book review, you may wish to emphasize this difference by differentiating between all publications and major publications (i.e. research papers, review articles, editorials). You may also wish to differentiate between publications and presentations in primary care venues versus non-primary care venues.

If the department has established particular research-related expectations or an agenda, it is important to keep statistics relevant to those criteria. Thus, our department established expectations that all faculty be involved in scholarship, and that faculty submit manuscripts for publication each year (one per year for part-time faculty and two per year for full-time faculty). Following such statistics is helpful in assessing progress. In addition, progress towards research agendas needs to be assessed as well. Thus, we followed the amount of scholarship directed at Hispanic issues in terms of the number of research studies, and the number of grants and their funding rate.

Goals of Scholarship

Evaluation is most helpful when focused on specific goals. Individual measures of productivity are then placed under these goals so that progress towards that goal can be assessed. Such benchmarks may be simple, such as having sufficient infrastructure support to cover salaries and pay for equipment upgrades. Benchmarks can also be lofty, such as changing practice; although changing practice may be an unrealistic (and unmeasurable) goal, communicating important ideas and changing paradigms may be more realistic. For example, assessing departmental reputation is measurable via such numbers as the number of invited presentations, visiting professorships, and trainees requesting positions. In San Antonio, we established three purposes of our research evaluation (*see* Tables 15.1–15.3):

1. to document excellence in research
2. to assist in resource management and efficiency
3. to document career progress for faculty.

Table 15.1 Scholarship Benchmarks Based on the Goal of Excellence in Research

Measure	Source
Number of Publications	CVs
Appointments/Elections	
editorial boards	CVs
officers of research organizations	CVs
National Research Committees	
national organizations	CVs
NIH study sections	CVs
Extramural Funding	
NIH ranking	NIH website
total amount ($)	Departmental records
distance to 10th place in rankings ($)[a]	NIH website
Number of Honors/Awards	CVs

[a] Relative to other departments of primary care.
CV: Curriculum vitae.
NIH: National Institutes of Health.

Table 15.2 Scholarship Benchmarks Based on the Goal of Resource Management and Efficiency

Measure	Source
Number of Manuscript Submissions Prior to Acceptance	CVs, faculty
Grant Proposals	
review outcome	
NIH scores	Pink sheets
status (funded, scored, not scored)	Pink sheets
resubmission rate	Research meetings
direct costs/staff involved in preparation	Grant proposals, Departmental grant preparation sheet
dollars submitted/dollars funded	Departmental records
Time Covered By Extramural Funding	
faculty	Departmental records
staff	Departmental records

CV: Curriculum vitae.

Table 15.3 Scholarship Benchmarks Based on the Goal of Career Progress for Faculty

Quarterly Focus/Measures	Source
Junior Faculty Submissions/Collaboration	
Manuscripts	
research, non-research	Junior faculty
authorship (solo, first author, seniority of co-authors)	Junior faculty
Grant Proposals	
training, research, career development	Junior faculty
collaborators	Junior faculty
Interdisciplinary Collaboration	
research projects	Faculty
manuscripts	Faculty
grant proposals	Faculty
Promotion and Tenure	
Success Rate	
assistant professor	P&T records
associate professor	P&T records
tenure	P&T records
Years to Promotion	
assistant professor	CVs
associate professor	CVs
Senior Faculty Impact	
Invited National Presentations	Senior faculty
Invited Publications	CVs
Circulation of Journals in which Publications Appeared	CVs, Internet
Citations	Web Of Science
Awards	CVs
Appointments	CVs
national committees	–
editorial boards	–
study sections	–

CV: Curriculum vitae.
P&T: Promotion and tenure.

Research excellence includes publications, research-related appointments and elections, service on national research committees, extramural funding, and honors and awards. Thus, using faculty curriculum vitae (CVs), departmental records, and the NIH website, we record the number of publications as well as appointments to editorial boards and election as officers of research organizations (e.g. the North American Primary Care Research Group (NAPCRG)). We record service activities on research committees of national research organizations as well as NIH study sections. We track total extramural funding, the department's NIH ranking, and the distance, in dollars, to the 10th place in NIH funding (NIH, 2002). Finally, the number of honors and awards is documented.

To assess our management of resources and research-related efficiency, we follow measures of research progress, manuscript submission, and funding. Thus, we use departmental records, CVs, and NIH "pink sheets" to track progress. In addition to ensuring that research projects are completed on time, and following the number of times a manuscript is submitted until accepted for publication, we record the amount of faculty and staff time covered by extramural funding. Grant proposals are also tracked closely, including their review outcomes (NIH scores, funding rate, rate of scored but not funded), their resubmission rate, and cost ratios. Thus, we track the ratio of direct costs received from funded grants to staff costs for grant preparation. In addition, we track the ratio of directs requested to directs received. Such measures allow us to assess how efficient we are in using resources and time in scholarly endeavors. Rhoades (2001) supports the inclusion of efficiency as a measure of productivity in academia.

Finally, using CVs, faculty surveys, promotion and tenure records, and the internet, we track career progress of faculty in four areas. To assess progress of junior faculty, we follow their submission rates of research and non-research manuscripts, and their authorship status on submissions; are they first author, solo author, and what is the seniority of co-authors? We track their grant submissions as to the type of grants submitted (research, training, career development), and their collaborations. A second area of career progress addressed is that of interdisciplinary collaboration. Thus, we track external faculty collaboration, both within the institution and outside, on research projects, manuscripts, and grant proposals. Promotion and tenure efforts are also tracked. We follow success rate for promotion to associate and full professor as well as for tenure. In addition, we track the years-to-promotion for both assistant and associate professor; for example, how many years does it take for an assistant professor to be promoted? Finally, we follow the impact that our senior faculty has on the discipline. Evidence of appointments to national committees, editorial boards, and study sections as well as receipt of awards is used. In addition, invitations to present at national meetings or to submit manuscripts are clear evidence of reputation. Other signs of impact include the citation rate of publications and the circulation of journals in which manuscripts are published.

Thus, more valuable than the individual measurements of productivity are measures geared to assessing progress towards departmental goals. This is the ultimate purpose of evaluation.

The Big Picture

The picture of evaluation presented above focuses upon how the research director can evaluate success in terms of research development within the department. However, the bigger picture deals with the extent to which research from the department impacts the discipline and healthcare system. For this, researchers and policy makers must communicate and share values. Researchers define "good research" as that which is logical, is respected by others, is directed at the discipline's paradigms, raises more questions, and has potential to influence others. Policy makers, however, define "good research" as relevant, applicable, understandable, available, and timely. Thus, researchers and policy makers often see research differently. If we researchers are to impact the discipline and the healthcare system, we must focus on producing research that meets the policy makers' definition. Thus, our studies must address research areas that are clearly relevant and applicable. We need to prepare understandable executive summaries and make them readily available to policy makers if they are to impact the decision making. Such activities will require a concerted effort to focus on communication with policy makers; it is unlikely that researchers will be able to change policy makers' views about "good research". The ultimate goal is, of course, for new investigators to choose important areas to research, and for new policy makers to train themselves in how to understand and use research (May, 1975).

But there can be a down side to such success (no matter whose definition is used). Departments with very successful research programs are at risk of injuring relations among faculty, creating "fiefdoms" and making clinician-teachers feel like second-class faculty. Teaching can be seen as an obligation as opposed to the opportunity of doing research. Researchers can develop an external orientation and may become a "traveling faculty", uninvolved in departmental issues. But it can also be damaging to the researchers themselves. Developing a Request for Applications (RFA) mentality may cause researchers to focus on the research area "du jour" rather than on an area of importance or in which they have particular talents. Very successful programs are particularly at risk of developing a soft money "house of cards", in which a sizable portion of the faculty and staff are dependent on grant money, and vulnerable to sudden loss of support (Eisenberg, 1986). These negative consequences to success must be addressed during the development process, rather than waiting until research success has already changed the faculty.

Synthesis

This section has emphasized the long-term development of departmental scholarship. Beginning with the establishment of a research culture, founded on trust and energized through its synergy, the research endeavor can be promoted through a smorgasbord of interventions and events tailored to each departmental/residency environment, but ultimately must include mentors, financial resources, and research laboratories. Finally, evaluation is the only means by which to follow your progress and to make corrections early. Using a variety of measures, evaluation should be goal based, and focused on the desired direction of the department and of individual faculty. However, ultimately, the goal of all research is to have an impact on colleagues and decision makers, while avoiding the potential negative consequences of success.

To this point, we have focused on the traditional approach to research development, based on traditional assumptions and using traditional interventions. Section IV questions these assumptions at both the departmental and individual levels, and suggests non-traditional approaches to research development.

Section IV

Building Research within the Complex Adaptive Departmental System

## Chapter 16

Complex Adaptive Systems

Vignette

L.M. understood that he was a small cog in a larger research machine; in fact, his productivity was still low, but he was independently productive thanks to a couple of small grants. As the senior faculty began to publish in *JAMA* and succeed in landing a couple of ROIs, the visibility of the department soared, both within the institution and externally. Researchers in other departments were more enthusiastic about collaborating with him and National Institutes of Health (NIH) project officers commented on the work of the senior faculty, suggesting the positives of including them as consultants on grants. It suddenly occurred to him that the interconnectedness and multilevel effects within the department meant that success of the department and its research teams led to trickle-down effects that reached even the least productive investigator.

Previous research has looked at building research capacity at both the departmental and individual levels. However, such studies seeking to model research productivity have produced only moderate success at either the departmental/residency (Wagner *et al*, 1994; Mills *et al*, 1995; Katerndahl, 1996) or individual (Katerndahl, 1995; Ferrer and Katerndahl, 2002) levels. The problem with these studies (and the thinking that produced them) may be that they assume linear dynamics and a predictable response, even though much of nature is complex and behaves non-linearly.

As science begins to awaken to the reality of non-linear dynamics, non-linearity has been observed in everything from psychology (Barton, 1994; Guastello, 1995) and sociology (Dendrinos and Sonis, 1990) to physiology (Freeman, 1991) and organizational change (Dooley *et al*, 1995; Cheng and van de Ven, 1996; Dooley, 1997). Recently, medicine has identified non-linear patterns in such diverse areas as cardiac (West *et al*, 1985; Goldberger and West, 1987; Goldberger *et al*, 1988) and psychiatric (Yeragani *et al*, 1999) disease, as well as in the dynamics of families (Smith, 1994) and ambulatory practices (Miller *et al*, 1998). Such non-linear behavior is the calling card of complex adaptive systems, and suggests that maybe our failure to model research productivity and predictably intervene is due to the lack of recognition that academic departments and research units are, in reality, complex adaptive systems displaying non-linear behavior.

Principles of Complex Systems

Complex adaptive systems consist of multiple, interacting agents capable of adaptive behavior (*see* Appendix 2). There are seven basic elements to complex systems – four properties and three mechanisms. Based upon these properties and mechanisms, we can describe a complex system through its characteristics. All of these properties, mechanisms, and characteristics apply to academic departments and ultimately to their research productivity.

The first property of complex systems is that agents tend to aggregate into functional units. Second, complex systems are maintained by the flows that occur between agents within the system. Such flows can be any commodities that can be exchanged, from food and energy to money and information. Third, complex systems are characterized by their diversity; their adaptive abilities depend upon it. Finally, complex systems display non-linearity in their behavior. Non-linearity means that the behavior of the system is not proportional to the sum of the behaviors of its agents; the amount of input is not proportional to the amount of output. These properties depend upon three basic mechanisms. First, agents within complex systems have tags; complex systems depend upon these recognition tags to form aggregates from its diverse agents. Second, complex systems use internal models or sets of rules to anticipate and react in standardized ways. The final mechanism is the use of building blocks. Complex systems decompose scenes into components, and recombine them in novel ways (Holland, 1995).

It is a small step to realize that academic departments and their research divisions display these properties and mechanisms, thus satisfying the definition of complex adaptive systems. Departments and divisions are composed of multiple faculty members (agents) with diverse skills and experience, distinguished by their roles, skills, and positions (tags). Such faculty members aggregate into clinical and research teams within divisions, differentially exchanging information (flows). By combining their standardized approaches to problems (internal models) with novel combinations of actions and agents (building blocks), they display non-linear behavior, in which group performance is greater than that of individual faculty members. Thus, multidisciplinary research teams combine standard research approaches to problems with each member's unique research tradition to produce investigations beyond the capability of its individual members.

Thus, we can describe the complex system of an academic department producing research by its characteristics. First, the research division can be described by its components, its researchers. Second, the research unit can be described by its interconnectedness and interdependence. These concepts, though related, are different. Interconnectedness relates to flows between agents such as information exchange between researchers, while interdependence relates to collaborations in which one faculty member's productivity is affected by another's, leading to non-linearity. Interconnectedness impacts the system's resistance to attack and its capacity for complexity. Weakly connected systems have greater capacity for complexity than fully connected systems, because they have greater capacity for combining novel patterns. However, fully connected systems are less vulnerable to attack; loss of any agent will have minimal effect on information exchange (Bar-Yam, 1997). Studies of networks suggest that all networks display similar properties and may grow via similar mechanisms. They tend to follow the "80/20 rule" in which 20% of the nodes receive 80% of the connections. In fact, networks follow a power law, in which the distribution of the frequency of nodes versus the numbers of connections follows the same pattern from network to network. This can be explained if networks continue to grow and if additional nodes connect preferentially to nodes with more connections or with greater fitness (Barabasi, 2003). In addition, the degree of connectedness has an impact on the system's dynamics; poorly connected systems display periodic dynamics, highly connected systems display chaotic dynamics, and critical systems with their power law dynamics have intermediate numbers of connections (Kauffman, 1993). Third, researchers will use their interactions and flows of funding and information to self-organize into interdependent research teams (Bar-Yam, 1997), capable of using their diverse backgrounds and skills to go beyond their individual abilities. This new synergistic behavior is called "emergence" and results in non-linearity. Finally, complex research units will display complex behaviors such as non-linear dynamics and co-evolution (Bar-Yam, 1997). While linear behavior is cyclic and predictable in both path and response to intervention, due to strong attractors limiting the possible behavior, non-linear behavior is neither cyclic nor predictable. Chaotic dynamics, though also dependent upon attractors, is sensitive to small initial changes in position (sensitivity to initial conditions). Thus, although chaotic systems follow predictable patterns over time due to their attractors, the specific paths they follow are unpredictable due to this sensitivity to initial conditions. Ultimately, this means that chaotic systems respond unpredictably to intervention; a small well-timed intervention may have a large effect, while a large intervention may have a small effect. The ultimate in non-linearity is seen in random dynamics, in which not only path and pattern, but response to intervention are unpredictable due to both sensitivity to initial conditions and the lack of attractors. But even within random systems, trends can be seen. Thus, true randomness (white noise), in which each point is totally independent of its predecessors, differs from power law criticality (pink noise), in which there is a trend over time for the system to return to previous values through periodic "avalanches" of behavior brought on by, among several possible mechanisms (Morel and Ramanujam, 1999), the varied thresholds or predilections of interconnected agents to react to ongoing stressors. Such critical or complex dynamics develop through self-organization at the interface between chaotic and periodic dynamics, and are inherently unstable (Morrison, 1991). In fact, as Figure 16.1 demonstrates, non-linear systems can display all of these dynamic patterns, depending upon the resources or constraints operating in the system. Co-evolution, on the other hand, takes the system's complex dynamics a step further, suggesting that the system's behavior must be interpreted based on its relationships with other external systems. Thus, interacting complex systems tend to increase their mutual complexity over time in order to survive (Bar-Yam, 1997); such interaction with its environment alters a system's fitness landscape as discussed below (Kauffman, 1993). Thus, a research team's behavior may reflect its relationship to other research teams within the department (perhaps because one researcher is part of both teams, or because they must share resources), or a research unit's behavior may be affected by the behavior of research units in other departments or institutions (as we compete for the same NIH funding).

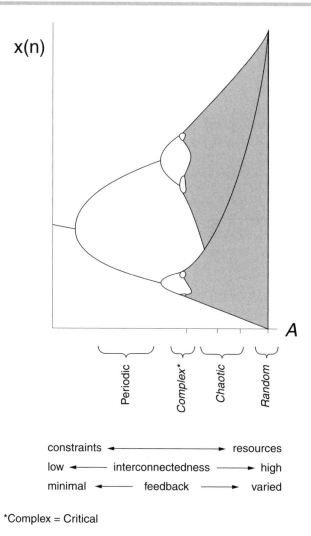

*Complex = Critical

Figure 16.1 Changing Dynamics of Chaotic Systems (Adapted from Liebovitch, 1998).

Complex systems live within a fitness landscape, a spatial description of a system's possible states, in which the basic terrain is punctuated by peaks in fitness, varying in quantity, height of fitness, and size of its base (its basin of attraction). Fitness landscapes are dependent upon the system's interconnectedness, but deformed by its environment and co-evolution. With no interconnections, the landscape consists of a single, high-fitness peak, but as interconnectedness increases, so does the number of local peaks while their individual fitness drops. Similarly, as the number of agents in a system increases, the expected fitness of local peaks decreases, and the number of steps needed to find a higher-fitness peak increases. Overall, system catastrophes can generally be avoided if the interconnectedness stays small, as the number of agents rises because the peaks with the highest fitness also have the largest basins of attraction (Kauffman, 1993). Thus, the fitness or effectiveness of a research team is dependent upon its size, its interconnections among team members, its environment within the department and institution, and its co-evolution over time.

Overall system complexity is based on the number of possible states, and is difficult to measure, but can be estimated relatively based on the system's error rate (more complex systems make more errors), and upon its informational content. There are three characteristics of system complexity that are relevant to research productivity. First, total system complexity for binary decisions is the product of output complexity and two raised to the power of the input complexity:

$$\text{Total complexity} = (\text{Output complexity}) \times 2^{(\text{Input complexity})}$$

Thus, the system complexity is far more dependent upon the complexity of the input than the complexity of the output. Second, in complex versus random or ballistic systems, as the scale (level of magnification in space or time) changes, so does the apparent complexity (*see* the complexity profile in Figure 16.2). Thus, whereas complexity does not change at all in ballistic systems, and transitions rapidly from maximal to zero in random systems, in complex systems complexity decreases as the scale becomes coarser, the curvature of the decline being dependent upon the resources available within the system. Finally, in trying to understand complex systems, we are limited by our own complexity. If the human brain has a capacity of between 10^{10} and 10^{11} bits of information, then a human cannot fully comprehend a system and its behavior if the system's complexity is more than 10^{11} bits. This may have important implications for our ability to understand the behavior within our own complex systems (Bar-Yam, 1997).

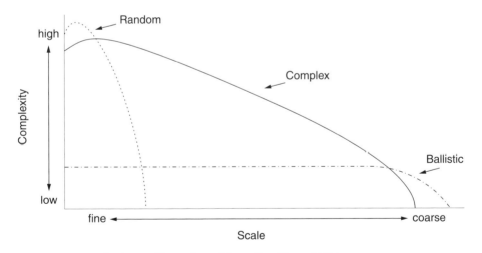

Figure 16.2 Complexity Profile (Adapted from Bar-Yam, 2002).

Synthesis

Complex adaptive systems are everywhere because their characteristics are inherent to living systems . . . including those of research units. Whether at the level of the researcher, the team, or the department, the research director must recognize the complex nature of its scholarship. This implies that small interventions may produce dramatic effects, while large, costly interventions may go unnoticed by the system. This also implies that the effect of interventions may ripple through the system in unexpected ways with untoward results. The research director must be prepared for these eventualities, must look for those leverage points, and must seek to support adaptation through emergence in an ever-changing fitness landscape.

## Chapter 17

Evidence for Multilevel Complexity in Research Programs

Vignette

L.M.'s mentor had made it clear; it was time for him to move to a higher level of productivity. First, the days of simple encouragement were over. He was to seek out situations in which he would receive a variety of feedback from a variety of sources, a mixture of positive and negative, weak and strong, comments. Second, his focus on "lone wolf" projects needed to evolve into multidisciplinary, collaborative studies in which he served in a variety of roles. Finally, he had concentrated on generating publications to build his track record; now his mentor wanted him to focus on understanding his area of research and its methods. The publications were no longer to be the focus; they would come.

Because activity at a fine scale can explain activity at a coarse scale, to fully understand a complex system such as an academic department requires a multiscale (individual-collaboration-department) description (Bar-Yam, 1997; Rhoades, 2001). From the annual collection of data on scholarly productivity among the faculty in San Antonio, scholarly activity time series datasets were constructed for each faculty member, for stable collaborations, and for the department as a whole. Nine measures of scholarship were used: three measures of activity (numbers of research studies and non-research projects, and research progress as measured by the number of stages completed), three measures of scholarship submissions (publication, presentation, and funding), and three measures of outcome (publications, national/international presentations, and funded grants). Cluster analysis was applied to data from individual faculty members, with at least 15 years of measurements to categorize them as displaying either low productivity, moderate productivity, or high productivity. This resulted in two faculty members in the low-productivity cluster, two faculty members in the moderate-productivity cluster, one faculty member in the high-productivity cluster, and one faculty member as transitional between low productivity during the first half and moderate productivity during the second half. In addition, inter-faculty collaborations active over at least three consecutive years on more than one project were identified. In order to determine the dynamics of scholarship at the individual and departmental levels, a series of analyses were applied which

1. assessed whether linear modeling could explain the pattern
2. assessed the degree of sensitivity to initial conditions in the data
3. assessed whether an attractor was present.

These three determinations could then suggest whether the underlying dynamics were periodic, chaotic, or random. Because some collaborations lasted only a few years, dynamics could not be assessed; instead, variability of scholarship across individuals, collaborations, and the department was used as an estimate of complexity and plotted as a complexity profile. In addition, social network analysis was applied to the department-wide collaboration network. Although the results may only apply to the department in San Antonio, they may in fact apply generally to scholarly activity in departments with established programs of scholarship.

Dynamics of Scholarship among Individual Faculty

Table 17.1 presents the results of the analyses of dynamics for all nine measures of scholarly activity for all six faculty (Katerndahl and McDaniel, 2003). Low productivity faculty generally displayed periodic dynamics. Analysis of the variability of their scholarship as measured by coefficients of variation (COV) showed that the variability of their submissions and outcomes was greater than that of their scholarly activity. Thus, low productivity faculty displayed periodic dynamics and were more consistent in their scholarly activity than in their submissions. The predominance of periodicity may suggest that low-productivity faculty have high expectations or few resources, that they focus more on outcomes than process, that they have few collaborative relationships, or that there is a close coupling of action and outcome. The implication of periodic dynamics is that scholarship in low-productivity faculty should be predictable and amenable to intervention; previous work supports the impact of fellowship/ research training and educational interventions on future productivity in terms of presentations, publications, and grants (Hekelman *et al*, 1995a; Taylor *et al*, 2001; Ferrer and Katerndahl, 2002). Moderately productive faculty showed more chaotic and white-noise random patterns, particularly in their scholarly activity. The chaotic processes may result from feedback of variable strength and direction, as well as from situations in which there are few constraints but adequate resources. A high degree of collaboration can also produce chaotic dynamics. In addition, because chaotic systems involve a lag between action and outcome, success requires a commitment to process rather than outcome. Besides the chaos observed in moderately productive faculty, white noise randomness was also seen, suggesting that current productivity was independent of prior productivity, but may also represent high dimensional chaos. In either case, chaotic and random dynamics suggest that response to intervention will be unpredictable. The dynamics of the transitional faculty member suggest that, when moving from low to moderate productivity, the first measures that change dynamics are non-research activity, presentations, and grants. The high-productivity faculty member generally displayed pink-noise randomness or criticality. Such dynamics occur when components interact and monitor progress via information exchange, altering behavior. Such systems display creativity and organization, and may reflect careful collaboration, time saturation, and competing demands (Jaen *et al*, 1994), leading to ongoing self-renewal (Overman, 1996). This may explain previous work noting correlation between scholarly outcomes and both service and other forms of scholarship (Taylor *et al*, 2001; Ferrer and Katerndahl, 2002). Such dynamics suggest unpredictable response to intervention. Assessment of

Table 17.1 Assessment of Individual and Departmental Dynamic Patterns in Time Series Data (Katerndahl, 2000b; Katerndahl and McDaniel, 2003)

Measure	Low Productivity		Transitional	Moderate Productivity		High Productivity	Department
	L-1	L-2		M-1	M-2		
Activity							
Research studies	Periodic[b]	Periodic[b]	Periodic	Uncertain	Chaotic	Random (P)	Periodic[b]
Non-research projects	Periodic	Chaotic[b]	Random (P)	Random (P)	Random (W)[b]	Random (P)	Chaotic[b]
Total progress[a]	Uncertain	Uncertain	Random (W)[b]	Random (B)	Random (W)	Random (P)[b]	Random (P)
Submissions							
Publications	Periodic	Uncertain	Periodic	Periodic	Random (W)	Random (P)	Uncertain
Presentations	Periodic	Uncertain	Random (W)[b]	Random (W)	Random[b]	Periodic	Periodic[b]
Grants	Fixed	Fixed	Chaotic[b]	Chaotic	Chaotic	Chaotic[b]	Random (P)
Outcomes							
Publications	Periodic	Uncertain	Random (P)[b]	Chaotic	Chaotic	Random (P)	Periodic[b]
Presentations	Periodic	Chaotic	Random (W)[b]	Random (W)	Random[b]	Random (P)	Periodic
Funded grants	Fixed	Fixed	Uncertain	Random (W)	Periodic	Chaotic[b]	Random (P)

[a] Total progress in research stages completed.
[b] Consistent on all analyses (ARIMA, Lyapunov, Correlation Saturation, Surrogate Testing).
W: White noise.
P: Pink noise.
B: Brown noise.

variability among moderate- and high-productivity faculty showed that variability in research progress was greater than other activity, and that variability in
funding was greater than other outcomes or submissions. Thus, moderate- and
high-productivity faculty maintain consistency in the numbers of active projects
and submissions, but cannot ensure consistency in total research progress or
funding.

Across clusters, research progress displayed randomness, only differing in the
type of noise, and grant submissions generally displayed chaotic dynamics.
However, clear trends from periodic to chaotic to random dynamics as productivity increased were observed for research and non-research activity, publication
submissions, and both publication and presentation outcomes, suggesting that as
faculty move from low to high productivity, their non-linearity increases, and
that non-linearity may be important to that transition. This may be consistent
with the observation that the COV for publications among chiropractic faculty
was larger among full professors than among assistant and associate professors
(Marchiori *et al*, 1998). If dynamics are viewed on a continuum (*see* Figure 16.1),
then as productivity increases, so does dimensionality. Based on computed
variability, non-research activity showed greater variability than did research
activity. This agrees with previous observations that research activity follows
patterns that are more predictable than those of non-research activity, at both the
individual (Ferrer and Katerndahl, 2002) and departmental levels (Katerndahl,
1996). However, variability in submissions was similar to that of outcomes for
both presentations and publications; and variability in research progress was
similar across all faculty.

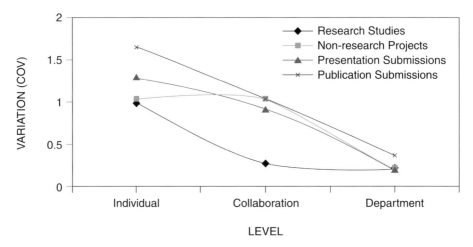

Figure 17.1 Comparison of Variation in Measures of Scholarly Activity Across Levels.

Dynamics of Scholarship in Research Collaborations

Figure 17.1 shows the change in variability in four measures of scholarship as the scale changes from the individual to collaboration to departmental level. As expected, variability decreases as scale increases. The interesting observation is the pattern of these changes and the concavity of the curves. While the curves for submissions of presentations and publications show a linear change, those for research and non-research activity are curvilinear, reflecting differences in the constraints and resources available to collaborations for these activities. The concave curve for research activity indicates that constraints are at work in the research collaboration. On the other hand, the convex curve for non-research activity suggests the paucity of constraints in non-research collaboration. Comparing the change in dynamics of moderate- and high-productivity faculty as we move to a departmental focus, we see that the randomness often seen in submissions at the individual level leads to periodicity at the departmental level. Similarly, the chaos and randomness of research activity at the individual level lead to periodicity at the departmental level. These observations are consistent with the complexity profile. The randomness of non-research activity at the individual level leads to chaos at the departmental level, reinforcing the lack of constraints at work at all levels for non-research activity.

Constructing the departmental collaborative networks for research (*see* Figure 17.2) and non-research activity provided further insights into the impact of collaboration on departmental scholarship. Table 17.2 shows the results of social network analysis conducted on collaborations within the department in 1998 and 2003. Although the cohesion scores suggest that there is significant networking within the department, the research cohesion dropped from 1998 to 2003, but it remained higher than non-research cohesion. Similarly, research centrality dropped, but not to non-research levels. These analyses suggest that research became less dominated by a few highly connected researchers; non-research in the department is less a product of collaboration than is research. The density of the research network increased (with a greater number of possible collaborations actually occurring). With network variability and adaptiveness maximized at a density of 0.5, research density is nearly maximized. The average number of research collaborations was 3.94 in 2003. This is considerably less than the scholarly collaborations on biomedical publications that Newman (2001) found from 1995 to 1999, which showed an average of 14.8–18.1 collaborations per author. However, his figures were based on publications only, included non-research publications, and covered five years. Finally, the average numbers of steps needed to reach other researchers within the department remained constant (around 2.25), less than that for non-research. Newman (2004) found that the average distance among biomedical authors was 4.4–4.6; this difference may again be due to differences in methods and setting. The degree of clustering within the department (clustering coefficient) was 0.501 in 2003 research, considerably larger than the clustering coefficients for medicine found by Newman (2004) of 0.066–0.072, but similar to those of both physics and computer science, suggesting strong collaborative groups within the department. Such mature networks develop a log–log relationship between the numbers of agents and the numbers of connections, suggesting the power law relationship that is characteristic of self-organized criticality. Thus, in fully mature networks,

80% of the connections center around 20% of the nodes (Barabasi, 2003). In our department, 20% of the researchers produced 50% of the research activity. These mature networks with their power laws form through continuous growth, in which new agents (collaborators) are added preferentially to connect with collaborators with either many other collaborations, or high productivity (Barabasi, 2003). Comparing the change in research collaborations from 1998 to 2003 in our department, high-productivity faculty showed more growth in collaborations than did highly collaborative faculty.

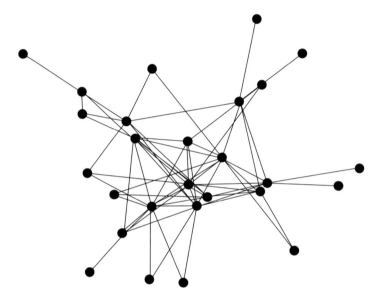

Figure 17.2 Departmental Research Collaboration Network.

Table 17.2 Results of Departmental Network Analysis

	1998	2003	
Measure	*Research*	*Research*	*Non-research*
Cohesion (connectedness)[a]	0.440	0.332	0.254
Density (connections:possible connections)[a]	0.560	0.617	0.118
Centrality (% centralization)[a]	0.353	0.240	0.118
Distance (no. of steps to reach others)	2.27	2.24	2.56

[a] Possible range = 0–1.

Another important factor in complex systems is the connections with other systems and their relationship with intra-system connectivity. If the product of the inter-departmental collaboration rate and the number of external departments involved is greater than the intra-departmental collaboration rate, then it will take the system a long time to reach its optimal fitness (Kauffman, 1993). In our department, as opposed to an average number of 2.58 intra-departmental research connections per researcher, researchers had an average of 0.346 external research connections with faculty in at least six other departments. Not only does a figure of 2.58 connections imply a maximum of five attractors involved, but it is within the 2–3 range expected to exhibit complex dynamics. In addition, Kauffman (1993) suggests that because 2.58 > 2.08 (0.346 × 6), all researchers involved should move quickly to maximize productivity.

Dynamics of Departmental Scholarship

Table 17.1 presents the dynamic patterns determined for all nine measures of scholarship at the departmental level (Katerndahl, 2000b). Compared with dynamics in productive individuals, overall dynamics at the departmental level tend to show more periodicity, as would be expected by the complexity profile. While research activity displayed periodic dynamics, non-research activity showed chaotic dynamics. Research progress as well as grant submissions and funding showed criticality. Non-grant submissions and outcomes generally displayed periodic dynamics. Although the initially assessed pattern for publication submissions could not be determined, when research and non-research submissions were assessed separately, research submissions displayed criticality, while non-research submissions showed periodic dynamics. These findings are consistent with those computed using data from nursing schools (Megel *et al*, 1988), in which the COV was larger for grants than it was for either publications or presentations. Thus, research studies and most submissions and outcomes display periodic dynamics, probably reflecting the presence of constraints and a focus on outcomes; these should be amenable to intervention. The criticality of research progress and grant activity implies competing demands, collaboration and monitoring, and an inability to intervene with a predictable response. Finally, the chaotic pattern of non-research activity may suggest that constraints are few, resources are sufficient, feedback is variable, and/or focus is on process rather than outcome. This is supported by work at both the individual and departmental levels showing that research activity is more predictable than non-research activity (Katerndahl, 1995, 1996). Although fewer non-research projects involve collaboration than do research projects (median 48% versus 72%), which should produce more non-linearity in research compared to non-research, the high degree of research constraints probably limits its dynamics.

Transitions between dynamics as activity moves to submission which, in turn, leads to outcome can sometimes be understood based on the continuum in dynamic patterns (*see* Figure 16.1). In the case of non-research, the transition is from chaos in activity to periodicity in submission for publication. This mirrors the exploration–exploitation transition seen in the innovative process in business (Cheng and van de Ven, 1996). In research, however, the transition is from periodicity in activity to criticality in submission for publication. This may represent the relaxation of constraints once the research data has been collected and analyzed. In either case, the transition from submission to outcome in both publications and presentations is strongly linked to periodicity, and may reflect the high acceptance rates of submissions for both publication (median = 74%) and presentation (median = 97%). In fact, submissions and acceptances are highly correlated for both publications (r_s = 0.91) and presentations (r_s = 0.66); there is no significant correlation between grant submissions and funding, both of which display criticality.

When looking at covariation of measures, two interesting patterns are seen. Figure 17.3 shows how change in research studies varies in relation to change in non-research projects. After a three-year period of growth in both during the department's developmental phase, these complementary forms of scholarship moved in opposite directions until the department entered its maintenance phase. Since entering this maintenance phase, change in research versus change in non-research has co-varied, either increasing or decreasing together, reflecting general support for scholarship within the department. On the other hand, the pattern of change in research versus non-research submissions for publication (*see* Figure 17.4) is one in which one (non-research) changes first, followed by the other (research) as the pair sequentially moves around the graph from quadrant to quadrant. This pattern is frequently seen in predator–prey relationships and reflects their interdependence. In other words, there is probably only so much time to support writing manuscripts, so when available time drops, non-research writing is the first to drop, followed by that of research. When time availability increases, it is easier to quickly resume non-research writing.

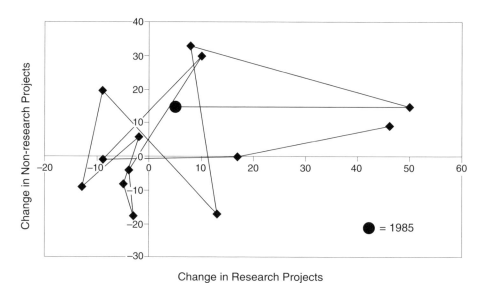

Figure 17.3 Change in Numbers of Research versus Non-research Projects (1985–1998).

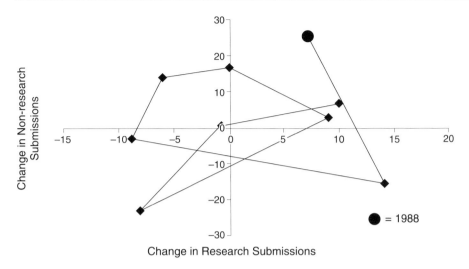

Figure 17.4 Change in Publication Submissions for Research versus Non-research Projects (1988–1996).

Synthesis

Although this in-depth case study focuses on the complexity and dynamics of scholarship in one department, there is a general message embedded within. This evidence attests to the validity of viewing research units as complex systems with all of their inherent characteristics and behavior. Although the specific dynamics exhibited in a particular measure by another researcher in another department may differ from what is reported here, the pattern of increasing non-linearity and tuning to criticality as individual productivity increases is probably generalizable, as is the decreasing apparent complexity with increasing scale; departments should behave more predictably than their component research teams or individuals. Such generalizations have important implications for the research director.

## Chapter 18

Research Development Based upon the Recognition of Complexity

Vignette

K.N. had waited and watched, studying the fluctuations of the department's productivity. She had a small pot of research funds from her Health Resources and Services Administration (HRSA) grant and had some uncommitted research assistant time. She wanted to boost research output, but had watched as fatigue and clinical commitments had drained the research faculty, leading to a "steady state" level of productivity. But she had studied closely a time in the department five years ago when a sudden surge in new research had occurred after a similar period of steady state dynamics. The surge had followed a departmental lecture from a visiting professor concerning a new paradigm of practice. Current frustration among faculty centered around mental health carve-outs. K.N. decided to arrange for a new faculty member in psychiatry to make a couple of presentations concerning his work, centering around the need for a new system of mental health classification for primary care. She would then hold a research retreat to allow these new ideas to percolate among the faculty, offering her pilot funds and research assistant time as support. If the timing was right, she would hopefully see a new surge in productivity and enthusiasm.

It is clear from the above multiscale description of one academic department with an established program of scholarship that, if representative, research programs function as non-linear complex systems. Consequently, intervention within such systems inherently produces unpredictable results; small interventions can lead to major changes (thanks to sensitivity to initial conditions), while large interventions can lead to only minor changes (thanks to attractors). Thus, as research director, responsible for the scholarly productivity of the department as well as the development of its individual researchers and collaborations, how can you use this insight for the benefit of researchers, collaborations, and the department?

There are several implications for intervention within a complex research program. First, acknowledge its inherent non-linearity and "rejoice" in it. Non-linear systems are capable of synergistic thought, and demonstrate both capacity for rapid adjustment and resistance to catastrophe. Chaotic dynamics are a sign of "health" – few constraints, adequate resources, a variety of feedback, and commitment to ideas and principles rather than outcomes (Cheng and van de Ven, 1996). Critical (pink noise) dynamics can be viewed as a self-renewal process (Overman, 1996). Maximal adaptability may be possible when a system is tuned to criticality (Morel and Ramanujam, 1999). Balanced between stable and unstable, between chaos and periodicity, critical systems are capable of rapid self-organization and emergence, the connection to higher-scale dynamics (*see* Figure 18.1). Such flexibility and balance may explain why most systems gravitate towards criticality (Kauffman, 1993). During times of change, organizations that embrace complexity fare better in the long run (Ashmos *et al*, 2000).

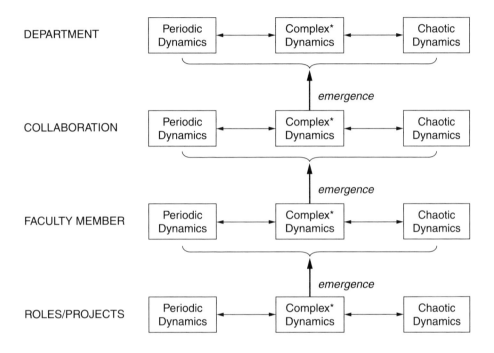

*Complex Dynamics = Critical Dynamics

Figure 18.1 Multiscale Emergence of Scholarship.

Second, know your system. On the one hand, an unrecognized lag between action and outcome may lead to non-linearity as we repeatedly intervene without allowing sufficient time for the first action to produce an effect (Senge, 1990). On the other hand, sensitivity to initial conditions implies that small, well-timed interventions can have dramatic effects. Thus, if we thoroughly know our complex program by longitudinally studying it and its response (Dooley, 1997), we may be able to identify when and how to optimally intervene, maximizing the probability of achieving the desired response from the system. However, both learning and sensemaking are different in non-linear systems than they are in predictable environments (McDaniel *et al*, 2003).

Third, reduce unnecessary complexity. When each health insurance company demands that its own unique claim form be used, that is unnecessary complexity. Although complexity within systems is associated with adaptability and fitness, unnecessary complexity only impairs efficiency and increases error. Reducing unnecessary complexity requires a thorough knowledge of the system and should focus on sources of input complexity to maximize effect.

Fourth, whole system intervention may be necessary. Within complex inter-connected systems, an intervention at one site may cascade throughout the entire system in unanticipated ways. "Every effort to promote productivity has the potential to trigger counterproductive responses and outcomes" (Rhoades, 2001). Unfortunately, most studies continue to take a reductionism approach, studying only a portion of the system and how it responds, and then generalizing to the rest of the system. Systems theory dictates that, before any intervention is implemented, its impact on the entire system must be considered. Thus, inter-ventions in complex systems must be viewed as system-wide interventions.

Fifth, consider connections. The process of self-organization is dependent upon the number of agents, the interactions among agents, and the flow of information and funds between them. Large numbers of agents predispose to self-organization, and the interactions between units may lead to increasing complex-ity (Morel and Ramanujam, 1999). A system's dynamics may be a product of its interconnectedness; two or fewer connections per agent leads to periodicity, while between two and three connections leads to criticality, and more than three connections leads to chaos (Kauffman, 1993). Critical systems rely upon their interconnectedness, continuous self-monitoring, and variable thresholds for reactivity to produce pink noise dynamics (Sharp and Priesmeyer, 1995). It is easier, and probably just as effective, to work on improving the performance of the poorest-functioning unit within a system than to set an ill-defined productiv-ity goal for the system. In addition, as the productivity of any unit changes within the system, so too does the productivity of the other interconnected units (Morel and Ramanujam, 1999). Interconnectedness can be utilized; numbers of connec-tions can be encouraged or restricted; interventions can focus on one part and then allowed to percolate throughout the system.

Sixth, it is possible to change dynamics. Although the use of "weak chaos" and "anti-noise" methods have been used to keep chaotic systems from slipping into periodicity and to change the color of noise, such methods have had limited success and the system's response is still unpredictable (Christini *et al*, 1996). However, non-linear systems can display different dynamics depending upon the complexity of the system's environment, as measured by A (*see* Figure 16.1). When A is low, the environment is stable and periodic dynamics prevail; when A is high, the environment is energetic, and chaotic and random dynamics are seen. Thus, it is possible to change the dynamics of a non-linear system by changing the complexity of the environment in terms of constraints, decision making, feed-back, connectedness, and resources. In reality, productive yet innovative systems depend upon a variety of dynamics. Exploration (chaotic dynamics) without exploitation (periodic dynamics) is unproductive, while exploitation without sufficient exploration is destructive over the long term (Dooley, 1997). These approaches are further supported by Rhoades (2001) who advocated focusing on encouragement of productivity and minimizing controls.

Finally, attractors can be used to manipulate system behavior. Because attractors dictate system behavior, changing attractors, though difficult, will result in changes in system behavior. While "hammering" is a method of attacking an attractor and thus shocking the system, it leads to unpredictable results. "Wedging", on the other hand, seeks to gently move an attractor in a desired direction through progressive nudging. Similarly, "joining" gently influ-ences a system by reinforcing desired attractors while weakening negative attractors (Miller *et al*, 1998). These gentle methods are more likely to succeed than "hammering" in producing a desired change.

How do these possible interventions play out in the fostering of scholarship within individual faculty members and their collaborative groups? How can these interventions be applied to non-linear departments? Table 18.1 overleaf summarizes differences in general approaches, specific strategies, and evaluation when comparing traditional linear with non-linear perspectives. In general, the focus of linear perspectives is on exploitation and production of outcomes (publications and funded grants); competing demands have additive effects, resulting in a steady improvement in career trajectory. On the other hand, a non-linear perspective focuses on process and exploration, recognizing the potential multiplicative effects of competing demands, leading to irregular career trajectories. Specific strategies are single, well-defined interventions in linear models, focused on personal acquisition of new methods and sharing results, with programs of study tightly linking a series of studies. In non-linear models, strategies include the use of multiple unfocused interventions designed to enhance exploration and sense making. Finally, whereas evaluation from a linear perspective focuses on short-term individual success, evaluation from a non-linear perspective focuses on long-term group success (Rhoades, 2001). Realizing that results from the in-depth study of one department may not generalize to other departments, the reality that *all* departments are complex adaptive systems governed by the same mechanisms and properties suggests that these results should indeed apply generally, allowing us to make general recommendations.

Promoting Scholarship among Individual Faculty

The periodic dynamics seen for most measures in low-productivity faculty suggests that their scholarship should be predictable and amenable to intervention. This is supported by research associating fellowship or research training with future productivity, in presentations (Ferrer and Katerndahl, 2002), publications, and funded grants (Taylor *et al*, 2001; Ferrer and Katerndahl, 2002). In addition, Hekelman *et al* (1995a) found that an educational intervention could increase publications among low-productivity faculty. Thus, faculty development interventions may be successful in promoting scholarly outcomes among low-productivity faculty. For example, the number of research conferences attended by these faculty individuals predicts future scholarly productivity (Katerndahl, 2000a). In fact, non-linear approaches are probably not necessary to increase outcomes among faculty displaying periodicity; they should respond to simple interventions.

Moderately productive faculty displayed chaotic dynamics in research activity and submissions. Realizing that the white noise randomness they also exhibited may in fact represent high dimensional chaos (Brock *et al*, 1991), moderately productive faculty may rely heavily upon chaos. Intervention here will lead to unpredictable results. In fact, the need for intervention should be carefully considered, because such chaos may be quite healthy, indicating few constraints, adequate resources, and commitment to principles. If intervention is necessary, one option is to maximize the productivity, supporting its dynamics through provision of resources and varied feedback, while minimizing constraints. A second option is to use the system's sensitivity to initial conditions by either

Table 18.1 Approaches for Promoting Scholarly Productivity when Assuming Linear versus Non-linear Dynamics (Katerndahl and McDaniel, 2004)

Approach	Linear Setting	Non-linear Setting
General		
Purpose of scholarship	Exploitation	Exploration
Effect of competing demands	Additive	Multiplicative
Career trajectory	Slow, steady	Irregular
Strategies		
Interventions	Single, focused	Multiple, unfocused
Goal of support strategies	Learn new techniques	Sensemaking
Role of pilot studies	Assessing methods	Exploration
Relationships between studies	Tightly coupled	Loosely coupled
Value of conference attendance	Making presentations	Sensemaking
Use of continuing education	Learn new techniques	Sensemaking
Goal of collaboration	Personal contribution	Careful increasing of non-linearity
Goal of mentorship	How to behave	Confidence in abilities
Evaluation		
Assessing strategies	Short-term	Long-term
Assessing departmental success	Individual success	Group success

implementing multiple small whole-system interventions or by conducting in-depth study of the system to allow a small, well-timed intervention to alter its path. A final option is to change the dynamics. While it is possible to induce periodicity via institution of constraints or limitation of resources and feedback, such periodicity is likely to bring predictability at the cost of productivity. Although this imposition of constraints may explain the success of the North American Primary Care Research Group (NAPCRG) Grant Generating Project among experienced researchers (Campbell and Longo, 2002), such strategies are probably best reserved for short-term projects oriented toward skill development. Rather, it may be preferable in the long term to tune chaotic dynamics into criticality by altering its interconnections and/or its monitoring. For example, pruning unproductive collaborations may move the system into criticality.

Finally, high-productivity faculty tend to display the healthy signature of criticality, the balanced process of self-renewal. This may represent time saturation and a competing demands model (Jaen *et al*, 1994) applied to faculty time commitments. This concept is supported by the work of Fairweather (2002) who found that, across disciplines in academia, research and teaching productivity were inversely related; thus, the "triple threat" faculty member showing excellence in research, teaching, *and* service is no longer attainable. In such a situation, activities are so tightly coupled that alteration in one immediately affects other forms of scholarship. If intervention is needed, only multiple strategies using a variety of intertwined tactics implemented simultaneously have a chance of success (Eisenhardt, 1990). However, as with other well-functioning complex adaptive systems (Kauffman, 1993), high-productivity faculty function at or near the edge of chaos in a zone of criticality, an area capable of change and emergence (Sharp and Priesmeyer, 1995). Thus, if criticality is indeed the most desirable state, we can maximize productivity by providing resources, minimizing constraints, and supporting rapid, free exchange of information to assist in the system's self-monitoring process. An environment that provides ongoing support promotes the learning and sensemaking needed for non-linear scholars to be effective (Weick, 1995; McDaniel and Driebe, 2001).

Perhaps the most important insight in this study is that non-linearity increases with productivity. Although it is risky to make cause-and-effect conclusions, the fact is that as productivity increases, so does non-linearity. Thus, one approach to faculty development of researchers is to use strategies intended to move low-productivity faculty into non-linear patterns. Assuming that even systems that display periodicity are in fact complex systems capable of non-linearity, one approach is to reduce the constraints and promote adequacy of resources for the trained, low-productivity faculty member to increase the dimensionality as seen in Figure 16.1. Another possibility is that periodicity is a self-imposed phenomenon due to self-imposed constraints, such as lack of confidence, inadequately diverse feedback, and a focus on outcomes (e.g. promotion and tenure) rather than principles. This can be addressed by providing positive feedback initially to build confidence, followed by balanced positive and negative feedback to promote non-linearity as well as counseling on priorities. The emphasis on mentoring can address these strategies. These proposals are congruent with recommendations made previously (Bland and Schmitz, 1986; Megel *et al*, 1988; Collins, 1993; Taylor *et al*, 2001). In fact, Collins (1993) recommends the frequent use of small reinforcements; if they promote non-linearity, such reinforcements could have major effects. Finally, low-productivity faculty can be moved towards non-linearity by dispersing decision making through collaboration and mentorship. In fact, collaboration itself will naturally promote non-linearity; as interconnect-edness increases, so does non-linearity (Kauffman, 1993).

Thus, viewing researchers as complex systems within a complex system speaks to strategies for promoting scholarship. If faculty are committed to excellence in research, have adequate resources and collaborations but few constraints, and have developed organized systems co-ordinating their research, teaching, and service, then non-linear dynamics should characterize scholarship. Although whole-system approaches are most appropriate for moderate-to-high-productivity faculty, low-productivity faculty should respond to simple interventions in predictable ways, increasing their productivity. However, the ultimate goal of faculty development for low-productivity researchers should probably focus on strategies to promote non-linearity rather than simple interventions to increase scholarly output. The exception to this rule is the low-productivity faculty member who has no desire to become a productive researcher, but needs a few publications to secure promotion; simple, focused interventions in this case are appropriate.

Promoting Scholarship in Research Collaborations

For our department, dynamics at the level of collaborations are most constrained in its research activity, and least constrained in its non-research activity. Measures of cohesion, centrality, and density are higher for research than non-research activity; density is nearer to maximal for research than non-research activity. Although network growth is more dependent upon productivity than connectedness of the "hub", the 80/20 rule suggests that our departmental research network may be too small to exhibit the 80/20 rule or is not yet mature. These observations further suggest that, while the high cohesion and centrality may contribute to the constraints of research activity, the near optimal variability of its density may provide flexibility and ease constraints. Our clustering coefficient is more similar to that of "natural" sciences than medicine, suggesting tighter collaborative groups; this is probably good from a productivity standpoint. One strategy for promoting novelty in collaborative groups is via information exchange through shared membership, thus promoting co-evolution (Barabasi, 2003). The failure of the 80/20 rule may suggest that full research network maturity requires more than 15 years, or that 20% of clinical researchers cannot reach the 80% goal if expected to fully participate in teaching and patient care as well; to reach the 80% level, highly productive researchers may need to commit 80–90% of their time to research.

Network research, in general, suggests that mature collaborative networks function at the chaos–periodicity boundary, in the zone of complex behavior (Barabasi, 2003). Thus, intra-departmental collaboration tunes the departmental activity to the zone in which productivity, adaptability, and emergence are highest. Although this optimal state tends to develop naturally in all networks, the research director can consciously work to promote network development and maturity. First, although collaboration should not be forced or "required", it should be promoted via the provision of opportunities to share research interests and ideas, encouragement of non-scholarship collaboration (i.e. teaching, service), easing barriers that may constrain faculty collaboration (e.g. time), faculty development focused on being a productive collaborator, and policies that foster network growth. However, there is an optimal level of connectedness (2–3 collaborations per faculty according to Kauffman). In fact, mutualism only increases with increasing connectedness to a point, after which mutualism drops and competition rises, thus damaging the network (Kauffman, 1993). Thus, do not encourage excessive, uncommitted collaboration. To facilitate the growth of a healthy research network, mentors should encourage protégés to link up with departmental ''hub'' faculty; in fact, ''hub'' status may be desirable in mentors themselves. In addition, because healthy networks tend to grow modularly (Barabasi, 2003), recruitment priorities should be given to recruitment of productive research collaborative groups, rather than recruiting productive researchers and then trying to build research teams around them. A final consideration relevant to intra-departmental research networks deals with the impact of researcher loss. While mature networks are resistant to the effect of error and loss of its agents, loss of a ''hub'' researcher could be catastrophic to the network (Barabasi, 2003). Hence, it is advisable for research directors to identify those researchers who serve as departmental ''hubs'', and to take action to ensure that they do not leave the department; keep the ''hub'' faculty happy and supported.

Finally, the role of extra-departmental collaboration is important. Although collaboration with other disciplines has been advocated as a way of promoting faculty research productivity (Collins, 1993), and represents a source of new information and ideas (Barabasi, 2003), it must be balanced against intra-departmental collaboration. First, the number of other departments involved in collaboration should be kept low; as the number of departments increases, the amount of time to reach optimal fitness and fluctuations in fitness increase as well, but the average level of fitness decreases. In terms of the number of inter-departmental collaborations, the number of such collaborations should also be kept low; as they increase, the levels of fitness decrease. If such inter-departmental collaborations are kept low, then intra-departmental collaborations should also be kept low to maximize overall fitness levels. Although the specific formula for optimizing fitness may differ in human systems, the principles and potential dangers are probably true of all complex systems, and warrant our attention. Thus, limited external collaboration involving few external departments may be healthy up to point; although it may help individual researchers, external collaboration can be detrimental to the departmental research program if excessive.

Thus, viewing research collaborations and networks from a complexity standpoint suggests that, although non-research activity is more non-linear and relies less on collaborative involvement, research activity may require network influences to counter the periodicity-invoking constraints inherent in the research process. Healthy network development can be fostered and supported, recognizing that there is an optimal level of intra-departmental collaboration, with selective external collaboration to promote optimal fitness reached within a limited period of time.

Promoting Departmental Scholarship

As seen in Table 18.1, a non-linear perspective on promoting departmental scholarship has implications that sometimes contradict conventional wisdom. In general, the expectations that departmental leadership has for scholarship need to change. Scholarship needs to be viewed as exploratory, with the emphasis placed on the ideas it generates, and faculty career irregularity should be anticipated. Because the effects of competing demands are multiplicative, one of either two approaches should be taken: either you eliminate the potential catastrophic effects of competing demands by limiting faculty time for research to your most productive researchers, or you embrace the multiplicative effects and use them to reinforce each other, so teaching reinforces research and service in a common area. Interventions should be multiple, and should focus on supporting non-linearity and sensemaking. Although we have discussed ways of promoting individual and collaborative development, success is measured by long-term group productivity. The ultimate goal is the optimization of performance across levels (Rhoades, 2001).

Looking at the seven approaches to intervention in complex systems mentioned earlier, recognizing and embracing complexity is vital to long-term success. Embracing a complexity model, departmental research goals should reflect group success, an exploratory focus, and emphasize sensemaking. Studies of healthcare organizations in volatile environments show that those organizations that embrace complexity via pursuit of varied goals, use of varied strategies, participation of varied decision makers, and decentralization perform better over time than those taking a traditional approach (Ashmos *et al*, 2000). Thus, in the complex environment of competing demands, funding volatility, and information explosion, research programs need to use broad strategies to pursue varied goals with participation of the researchers involved. On the other hand, unnecessary complexity only adds constraints to the system and should be avoided.

In-depth knowledge of the system may enable you to identify leverage points where the system's sensitivity to initial conditions can enable you to intervene successfully with a minimum of effort. Thus, knowing the dynamics involved and the individual faculty "hubs" within the research network may allow you to focus interventions on a particular point in time or on a particular researcher and yet alter the entire system. On the other hand, the productivity of the entire department can be increased by targeting the least productive faculty (Morel and Ramanujam, 1999) who typically display periodic dynamics responsive to intervention.

Whole-system approaches can be essential when non-linear dynamics will diminish the effect of a single intervention, or when the entire system must change. For example, when instituting a research program where none previously existed, system-wide interventions such as policy changes affecting all faculty are critical to moving the system along.

Although we discussed the need to focus attention on development of a healthy network of research collaboration with limited external collaboration, connections are also relevant beyond those of individuals. Increasing the number of researchers increases the chance of self-organization and ultimately complexity; thus, there is probably a critical number of researchers necessary for self-organization to occur. Interconnectedness promotes non-linearity and enables teams to comprehend things more complex than any individual can. In addition, interconnectedness of projects and faculty roles can be important to producing the complex dynamics that promotes healthy scholarly dynamics at the next level, that of the researcher. Similarly, the interconnectedness of research teams encourages novelty and co-evolution, enabling non-linearity among them to develop, and emergence (or synergy) at the departmental level to be seen. Taken a step further, inter-departmental connectedness could promote emergence at the institutional level.

Recognizing the dynamical patterns of scholarship at the departmental level can be valuable to the research director. First, the definition of "healthy" dynamics may depend upon where the department is in its development, and upon its environment. When research is beginning, the research director should promote non-linearity and its commitment to process. When seeking to move the department to a "higher" level of excellence, critical dynamics may be necessary for the required emergence. Once the department has established its excellence and productivity, periodicity will serve to maximize that productivity. However, these recommendations are only true when the department exists within a stable environment; when the environment is volatile, critical dynamics are generally the best for enabling adaptation no matter where the department is in its development. Second, the desired dynamics also depend upon the targeted form of scholarship. For example, criticality is probably very healthy and not amenable to change, so the existence of such patterns seen in research progress as well as grant submissions and funding is probably a good sign, and should be supported via selective interconnections. Although it may be tempting to introduce constraints to impose predictable periodicity on the chaos of non-research activity, this is ill-conceived and likely to reduce overall productivity and true exploration. The periodic dynamics of research activity and submissions for publication and presentation suggest that these forms of scholarship are pre-dictable and amenable to intervention. However, it is important to remember that group interventions may produce group success without leading to productivity in every researcher; in fact, the low-productivity faculty with their linear dynamics will be most likely to respond. This may explain why the fitness of a group can be enhanced by focusing on improvement of the worst-performing agents (Morel and Ramanujam, 1999).

Finally, the use of attractors can be attempted if system-wide change is needed. For example, when trying to establish a research climate where none existed, the use of "joining" can be useful. While the "counterculture" attractor of family practice is downplayed, the positive attractors are emphasized. These include the attractors of "commitment to excellence" as demonstrated by the generation of new knowledge, "patient care focus" as demonstrated by linking research to good patient care, and "maintaining clinical competence" as demonstrated by evidence-based medicine (Katerndahl *et al*, 2002). A form of "hammering" is the introduction of a new attractor such as the hiring of a well-respected researcher whose presence will hopefully serve as a nidus for pro-research thought and idea generation, although such a response is not guaranteed. Thus, the use of attractors can be valuable in changing culture.

Synthesis

This section has focused on approaching research development through the lens of complexity. There is little doubt that departments and research programs have the properties and characteristics of complex adaptive systems. Analysis of one productive department supports this concept, suggesting that more productive faculty display more non-linearity than do less productive faculty, that research collaborations are more constrained than those of non-research, and that departments show a variety of dynamics depending upon the measure of scholarship. These findings suggest that research development needs to change its emphasis to a non-linear perspective, focusing on exploration rather than exploitation, sensemaking rather than skill acquisition, long-term group success rather than short-term individual success.

This ends our discussion about promoting scholarship at the individual and departmental levels based on linear and non-linear assumptions and approaches. But the department is not pursuing its scholarship in a vacuum; it is connected both spatially and temporally to the greater context of research within the discipline and beyond. As research director, you must be cognizant of this greater context, and cognizant of developments within the discipline and organized medicine.

Section V

The Future of Primary Care Research

Chapter 19

To Where We Head

Vignette

Resting on one's laurels is always comforting. K.N. had just left her annual meeting with the chair and he was singing her praises. After all, she had joined the department 10 years ago and had assumed the directorship of a non-existent research division. The division was now very successful in terms of publications and funding . . . and she was promoted to full professor! But there was also the gnawing feeling that she needed to start focusing on what would be her legacy, not just to the department, but to the discipline. True, she had published in a variety of journals and had served on a couple of national committees, but it didn't feel like much of a legacy. She resolved then and there that she would renew her commitment to taking her research passion to the next level, working to implement community and state programs, while leading national committees to change the discipline's attitudes as well as those of organized medicine.

The greater question is "to where are we collectively heading?" Do recent developments suggest that primary care will ultimately relinquish its research efforts and resume its teaching–care duality, dependent upon other disciplines for its knowledge base? Or have we researchers reached a point of synergy and complexity that may lead to emergence of a truly academic discipline, grounded in a commitment to the generation of new knowledge?

There is cause for concern. The level of research support is still poor, with Title VII funds perennially at risk and few researchers committing substantial time to research. Research fellowships continue to have unfilled slots (Elward *et al*, 1994) or slots filled by non-family practice physicians (Rodnick, 1999). Although the content of our research literature appears appropriate and reflects practice, the study designs continue to involve proportionally too little longitudinal and experimental research. The quality of the literature appears to be improving with increasingly more sophisticated statistical analyses being used. A major concern is that the research productivity of individual researchers continues to be low and, if anything, the research output of the discipline may be declining.

Tradition has dictated a certain disdain for research by family practitioners. Connelly *et al* (1990) reported that family physicians rarely used research, rating it as poorer than other information sources in terms of understandability and applicability. In fact, when offered free copies of the research journal *Archives of Family Medicine*, only 19,000 out of 100,000 family physicians requested a copy. When primary care physicians pursue an answer to a clinical question, 80% of the time an answer is found (Gorman and Helfand, 1995). Although resident family physicians generate at least one question per encounter on average, they seek immediate answers only 66% of the time. When they do seek answers, it is typically from a colleague or pocket reference (Ramos *et al*, 2003). If family practice faculty and residents seek answers online, 54% of questions are answered within 5–10 minutes. More importantly, 56% of these answers influenced the care of their current patient, and 70% would affect care of future patients (Schwartz *et al*, 2003). Compared with other primary care disciplines, family medicine lags behind in its use of research (Connelly *et al*, 1990), research requirements during residency training (Alguire *et al*, 1996), and the availability of research fellowships (Elward *et al*, 1994; Rodnick, 1999). Thus, there is not only cause for concern about trends in research productivity, but also about the value placed on research by members of the discipline.

Recent Developments

But there is also cause for some optimism. Several recent developments are encouraging, and suggest that the culture of family medicine may be changing, the prospect for support for research brightening. First, events may help to enhance national awareness of family medicine and primary care. In 1993, the Academic Family Medicine Organizations (AFMO) released a strategic plan for research in family medicine. It included recommendations for conducting family medicine research (i.e. targeting critical areas, fostering interdisciplinary collaboration), increasing research support (i.e. increasing funding opportunities, increasing family practice representation on study sections), and expanding research capacity (i.e. increasing the quantity of researchers, promoting research as a career) (Academic Family Medicine Organizations Steering Committee, 1993). Then, in 1996, the Institute of Medicine released its recommendations for primary care research. These included developing national databases and primary care datasets, developing standards for primary care data, endorsing the concept of practice-based research networks, and pushing for federal support of primary care research (Institute of Medicine, 1996). Finally, the American Academy of Family Physicians (AAFP) established its Center for Policy Studies in Family Practice and Primary Care (Green and Fryer, 1999). This center conducts and disseminates policy-relevant research, representing the discipline in Washington, providing a voice for primary care research in government venues. All of these developments have increased the visibility of primary care researchers.

Second, a couple of events have focused on development of our research capacity. The North American Primary Care Research Group (NAPCRG) appointed a Committee for Building Research Capacity. In addition to such activities as the Grant Generating Project and assessment of the current status of family medicine research, the committee defined what was involved in building capacity, recognizing that this entailed much more than grant support and training. In addition, this committee is particularly important because it brings together the leadership for family medicine research from various organizations on an annual basis. But perhaps an even more powerful event was the AAFP Research Initiative. Under this initiative, researchers were supported through external funding and the Advanced Research Training program, infrastructure was enhanced through practice-based research networks (PBRNs) support, and research enhancement was promoted through the establishment of three research centers and the pursuit of joint projects with managed care organizations (Scherger and Young, 1998). Judging by the ever-increasing attendance at the annual meetings of NAPCRG over the past five years, interest and involvement in research may be on the rise. These developments reinforced the idea that capacity building is a broad activity and requires broad support. In addition, in response to the AFMO Strategic Plan, the AAFP established a website dedicated to resources for family medicine researchers, FMResearch.org.

Third, events occurred to facilitate our ability to conduct and disseminate meaningful research. Recently, there has been development of relevant large databases, appropriate for addressing research questions important to family practice. These include the institution of annual collection of the National Ambulatory Medical Care Survey. To improve surveillance data in Europe, a computerized patient record based on ICD-10 and the International Classification of Primary Care (ICPC) has been proposed (Backer, 1993). Such databases greatly enhance our ability to conduct meaningful research. In addition, the Agency for Healthcare Research and Quality (AHRQ) has recently focused on infrastructure support for PBRNs. This, coupled with a growing appreciation by federal funding agencies for the value of practice-based networks, bodes well for the future of these research laboratories. Finally, in a landmark event, the major family medicine organizations joined forces to provide five years of support for the establishment of a new research-oriented journal, the *Annals of Family Medicine*. Not only is this development important for its provision of publication opportunities for research, but it is a key sign of an awareness by diverse groups of the need for and threat to primary care research, a sign that the culture of primary care may be changing.

Finally, there are developments that specifically focus on changing the anti-research culture of family practice. Although improved information retrieval has been advocated for family physicians for some time (Verhoeven *et al*, 1995), the development of the Family Practice Inquiries Network (FPIN) represents a major step in this process (Dickinson *et al*, 2000). More recently, the *American Family Physician* with its strong tradition of publication of qualitative reviews began to publish a group of patient-oriented evidence that matters (POEMs) in each issue of the journal. Coupling this with a growing requirement that its authors base their reviews on evidence rather than prior opinion suggests that the journal has shifted its focus. These developments suggest that the family practice culture itself is being targeted for change and that the discipline's leadership across the board recognizes the need for this change. Unfortunately, POEMs are still difficult to find. Over a six-month period in 1997, only 2.6% of articles published in 85 general medical journals were POEMs; most of these did not deal with common problems (Ebell *et al*, 1999).

In addition, prospects for other developments may also bode well for primary care research. First, the potential for research funding from the managed care sector is a growing possibility. Second, when and if true healthcare reform materializes in the United States, the resultant cost-effective, health-maximizing system would have to emphasize primary care as its basis; a national, specialty-based system could not, would not be either cost-effective or health maximizing. The Future of Family Medicine project includes "advancing research that supports the clinical decision making of family physicians and other primary care clinicians" as one of the priorities for healthcare reform (Future of Family

Medicine Project Leadership Committee, 2004). Thus, healthcare reform should bolster primary care research support.

Recommendations

If there are causes for concern but events targeted at aborting such disaster, where do we go from here? What must be done to promote the development of a strong research base for the discipline?

In 2000, NAPCRG's Committee for Building Research Capacity identified eight areas important to the concept of research capacity. These areas included linkages, infrastructure, training, reputation, publishing, culture, funding, and asking the right questions. Some key recommendations identified by the committee (*see* Box 19.1) included infrastructure support with protected research time, infrastructure funding, research positions, mentors, and research centers, training support for 2–3 years after fellowship with 50–80% protected research time, reputation promotion via inclusion of 3–4 family physicians on 5–10 study sections, and promotion of linkages via systematic networking among organizations and researchers (NAPCRG Committee on Building Research Capacity and AFMO Research Subcommittee, 2002).

Box 19.1 Concepts of Building Research Capacity (Adapted from NAPCRG Committee on Building Research Capacity and AFMO Research Subcommittee, 2002)

1. Linkages
   - Between researchers
   - Across practices
   - Between disciplines
   - Among networks, centers, and institutions
2. Infrastructure
   - Research centers
   - Protected time
   - Research positions
   - Grant management
   - Role models
3. Training
   - Research careers
   - Mentors
   - Advanced degrees
   - Skill development
   - Research fellowships
4. Reputation
   - Researchers on National Institutes of Health (NIH) study sections
   - Researchers on AHRQ study sections
   - Representation on federal agenda-setting conferences
5. Publication
6. Culture
   - Expectations for generation of new knowledge

- Valuing scholarship
- Instilling appreciation in residents and students
- Centers of research excellence
- Supporting development of independent investigators
7. Ask the right questions
   - Common practice or problem?
   - Practice-based perspective
   - Responsive to the needs of clinicians, policy makers, or funding agencies
8. Funding
   - AHRQ funding
   - NIH funding
   - Foundation funding
   - Alternative sources

In 2001, AFMO reviewed its 1993 recommendations and expanded them (see Table 19.1). Instead of limiting capacity building to promoting research conduct through fostering collaboration and the targeting of critical areas, research support through increased funding opportunities and primary care representation on study sections, and research capacity through increased numbers of researchers and research as a career, AFMO built on the areas identified by the Committee for Building Research Capacity and proposed recommendations under a broad range of areas relevant to building capacity. Thus, under "Infrastructure", the committee recommended the development of a clearinghouse for research-related information (i.e. information on family medicine researchers, funding opportunities, training opportunities, media resources, funded projects, databases, research instruments, publications), the creation of curricula for research administration and leadership, the compilation of successful models of research organizations, and the identification of a process for developing a family medicine research agenda. Under "Culture", the committee recommended increasing exposure of students and residents to positive role models, developing programs to enhance the perception of family medicine research, developing an expanded model of the domain of research activities for family physicians as well as promotion and tenure committees, increasing health disparities research, and increasing the numbers of researchers while facilitating participation in established training programs. Under "Training", the committee advocated characterization of fellowships, enhancement of research mentoring, enhancement of research skill development, facilitation of residency–fellowship transition, and development of minimum research knowledge standards for faculty and PBRN members. Under "Funding", the committee recommended cataloging resources for infrastructure funding, increasing grant submissions and awards for researchers, developing strategies for influencing funding agencies, working to build the Center for Primary Care Research within AHRQ, and developing research endowments. Under "Publications", the committee advocated the assurance of adequate, accessible venues for research, development of a list of family medicine research publications, and increase of manuscript submissions. Finally, the committee emphasized the need to evaluate relevant linkages, to demonstrate

Table 19.1 AFMO Recommendations for Building Research Capacity
(Adapted from AFMO, 2002)

Goals	Time Frame	Priority
Infrastructure		
A. Empower Groups to Take Responsibility for Tasks		
• Paid Staff		
• Defined Roles and Responsibilities		
• Acceptance by Participants		
B. Develop Clearinghouse for Materials	Short-term	High
• Names of Those Interested in Serving on Study Sections		
• Names of Those Who Can Serve as Spokespersons for Family Medicine		
• Funding Opportunities		
• Research Training Opportunities		
• Media Resources for Dissemination of Work		
• Links to Media Stories Regarding Family Medicine Research		
• Researchers' Biographies and Interests		
• Funded Grants and Projects		
• Publications by Family Medicine Researchers		
• Bibliography of Family Medicine Research		
• Research-oriented Clinical Information Systems		
• Datasets Appropriate for Family Medicine Research		
• Instruments to be Used in Family Medicine Research		
• Statistical Approaches for Primary Care		
• Qualitative Studies, Designs, and Analyses		
• Dissemination Opportunities		
• Special Interests and Capabilities of Departments		
• Links to Other Research-related Resources		
C. Create Research Administration Curricula	Short-term	
• Department Chairs		High
• Residency Directors		Low
• Research Directors		High
• Predoctoral Directors		Low
D. Compile Compendium of Models of Research Organizations	Short-term	Medium
• Developmental Stages		
• Gap Analysis		
– Other Primary Care Specialties	Short-term	High
– Family Medicine Departments	Short-term	High
– Family Practice Residencies	Long-term	Medium
– Practice-based Research Networks	Long-term	Medium
– Private Practices	Long-term	Medium
E. Process for Developing a Research Agenda	Short-term	Medium
Culture		
A. Expose Students and Residents to Models of Family Medicine Research	Short-term	Medium
• Medical students		
• Residents		

Table 19.1 (*cont.*)

Goals	Time Frame	Priority
B. Develop Programs to Increase the Perceived Value of Research		
• Develop Programs to Recognize Productivity in Teaching Centers and Practices	Long-term	High
• Social Marketing Issue	Short-term	High
C. Develop Expanded Model of Domain of Research Activities for Family Physicians and Promotion and Tenure Committees	Short-term	High
• Creation of New Knowledge		
• Synthesis of Existing Knowledge		
• Translation to Practices, Public, and Policymakers		
• Implementation in Practices and Health System		
• Evaluation		
• Organized Curiosity		
• Participatory Research		
D. Increase Role in Researching Health Disparities	Short-term	High
• Increase the Number of Minority Researchers		
• Better Define Research Issues		
• Improve Links to Funding Sources		
E. Develop Strategies to Increase the Numbers of Family Medicine Researchers	Long-term	High
F. Facilitate Participation in Established Research Training Programs	Short-term	Medium
• Robert Wood Johnson (RWJ) Foundation		
• K Awards		
• Minority Training Programs		
• Fellowships		
Training		
A. Characterize Fellowships Appropriate for Researchers	Short-term	Medium
B. Enhance Research Mentoring	Long-term	High
• Research Training Sessions at National Meetings		
• Explore Literature		
• Define/Develop Role		
• Identify Incentives		
C. Increase Expertise in Research Methods	Long-term	Medium
D. Facilitate Transition from Residency/Fellowship to Independent Researcher	Long-term	Medium
• Evaluate Models		
• Teach Negotiation Skills		
• Identify the Necessary Environment and Resources		
• Identify Leaders Who Will Mentor Residents and Develop Research Programs in Residencies		
E. Develop Minimal Standards for Required Research Knowledge for Faculty and PBRN Members	Long-term	High
F. Update Residency Curriculum Guidelines	Short-term	High

Table 19.1 (*cont.*)

Goals	Time Frame	Priority
Linkages		
• Working Group to Evaluate Existing and Required Linkages	Long-term	Medium
– Across Disciplines		
– Family Physicians to Community		
– Media and Practitioners		
– Research Community and Practice Community		
– Impact Practicing Physician Through AAFP Annual Assembly		
Funding		
A. Catalog Resources for Infrastructure Funding	Short-term	Medium
B. Increase Grant Submissions and Awards	Long-term	High
C. Develop Strategies to Influence Those Who Fund Research	Long-term	High
D. Billionize the Center for Primary Care Research Within AHRQ		
E. Develop Research Endowments		
Publication		
A. Adequate Venues to Publish Research that are Accessible to Others	Short-term	
B. Develop List of Family Medicine Research Publications		High
C. Increase Number and Type of Submissions for Publication		High
Reputation		
• Develop Strategies to Enhance Perceived Value of Research	Long-term	High
– Within Family of Family Medicine Researchers		
– Within Family of Family Medicine		
– Within Family of Healthcare		
– Within Communities		
– Within Congress and State Legislatures		
– Within Family of Funding Groups		
Right Questions		
• Demonstrate Importance of Framing Research Questions for Full Spectrum of Concerns, Symptoms, Diseases, and Multiple Conditions		

the importance of our research through the questions it addresses, and to enhance the perceived value of our research (Academic Family Medicine Organizations Research Subcommittee, 2002).

The Future of Family Medicine (FFM) project emphasized the ongoing need for primary care research, stating that all family physicians should be involved in the generation of new knowledge. The new model of family medicine proposed would include advanced information systems and a standardized electronic medical record, which would facilitate research. Practice-based research networks and departments of family medicine were cited for their roles in developing this interdisciplinary research base. In addition, the FFM project strongly advocated the need for federal research funding commensurate with that received by other disciplines; thus, AHRQ funding should be increased to at least $1 billion per year. In fact, a federal entity dedicated to research on whole-person health and healthcare should be established. Most importantly, we need to enhance the science of family medicine (Future of Family Medicine Project Leadership Committee, 2004).

These recommendations provide concrete guidelines for the discipline in charting its research future. But there are additional steps, which could further our efforts to improve the research base, improve the perception of primary care research, and develop a research culture within the discipline (Katerndahl *et al*, 2002; Parchman *et al*, 2003). In addition to previously mentioned recommendations that target improvement of our research base, we need to further expand our venues for presentation of research results by considering alternatives to paper journals, and to provide more research time for faculty. Some journals already provide online copies in addition to the paper version of the journal. Eventually, we need to expand our online journals to provide more venues for communication of research results. The old concept of the "triple threat" faculty member, involved and expert in teaching, research, and clinical care, must be abandoned in favor of a model that recognizes and values each faculty member's unique gifts, tailoring their commitments to their gifts (Healy, 1988). In addition to previously mentioned recommendations that target improvement in the perceived value of primary care research, we need to resist external assaults on the quality of our research and the care we provide (Block *et al*, 1996), as well as promoting research that documents the value of the principles upon which the discipline is based. Thus, when research critical of the quality of family practice care is published by other disciplines, a critical appraisal team needs to immediately address in writing the inevitable flaws inherent in the research (Katz *et al*, 1997). Conversely, the principles upon which family practice is based (AAFP, 2004) need to be the focus of more research, targeted for publication in our journals (as the recent issue on continuity of care in *Family Medicine*). Also, the AAFP Communications Division should develop strategies to publicize important family practice research findings in the media. Finally, in addition to previously mentioned recommendations that target the development of a research culture within the discipline, we need to seek additional ways to remold anti-research attitudes. Although promoting positive attitudes among residents is vital for long-term success, such a process is too slow for our immediate needs; we must actively attack anti-research attitudes among current practitioners. One approach would be to strengthen positive current attractors (provision of good patient care, practicality of information, competence) while de-emphasizing anti-intellectual fervor. In addition to emphasizing that competence depends upon incorporating research into practice, we need to reinforce the concept that research is part of good patient care. This can be approached through involvement in PBRNs (Weiss, 2000). We could encourage PBRN involvement via such programs as loan forgiveness or continuing medical education (CME) credit for PBRN involvement. We can emphasize the practical nature of our research through emphasis of practicality incorporated within all research publications and through inclusion of research findings within all CME presentations and review articles. Another approach that could be taken to remold attitudes would be to utilize "mainstreaming" concepts, which force individuals into activities that they eventually incorporate themselves. This approach would force practitioners into research participation as a condition for recertification. Although initially fought (undoubtedly), once involved, the practitioner would presumably come to see the value of research. Such requirements for recertification could include required PBRN participation, required research-related CME hours, or a required scholarly project.

Synthesis

Trends in family practice research over the past 10–20 years are concerning, but recent events suggest that the leadership recognizes the impending crisis and has taken steps to avert disaster. Recent recommendations, if implemented, could in fact turn the corner on primary care research, presenting renewed opportunities and renovating our anti-research culture into one that values inquiry and evidence, supports its development, and uses that research in its reform of healthcare. The director of research within the academic department or residency is in a position to encourage and develop individual researchers, to change anti-research attitudes within the next generation of family physicians, to remold anti-research attitudes among current practitioners within the community and PBRNs, and to promote primary care scholarship within their department or residency, their institution, and their discipline.

As research director, you must be involved in this re-invention of the discipline, involved in the community, involved in the local chapter of the AAFP, involved in the greater discipline. Emergence is not a product of mass; it is a fruit of interconnectedness. A single voice in a system poised in complex dynamics can ripple throughout, changing the system.

References

Academic Family Medicine Organization Steering Committee. *Strategic Plan Summary for Research in the Discipline of Family Practice*. Leawood, KS: Academic Family Medicine Organization Steering Committee, 1993.

Academic Family Medicine Organizations Research Subcommittee. *Building Research Capacity in Family Medicine: Draft of a Strategic Plan*. Leawood, KS: Academic Family Medicine Organization Research Subcommittee, 2002.

Aday LA, Quill BE. Framework for assessing practice-oriented scholarship in schools of public health. *J Public Health Manag Pract* 2000; 6:38–46.

Agency for Health Care Policy and Research (AHPCR). *Putting Research into Practice*. AHCPR no. PB 93-218584. Rockville, MD: AHCPR, 93-218584, 1993.

Alguire PC, Anderson WA, Albrecht RR, Poland GA. Resident research in internal medicine training programs. *Ann Intern Med* 1996; 124:321–8.

Almind G. Structures and strategies for general practice research in Denmark. *Scand J Prim Health Care* 1993; 11(suppl 2):8–9.

American Academy of Family Physicians. *Family Medicine* 2004. www.aafp.org/x6809.xml (accessed 4 October 2005).

American Geriatric Society Education Committee. Guideline for promotion of clinical educators in geriatric medicine. *J Am Geriatr Soc* 2002; 50:963–5.

American Medical Association. Future of family practice. *JAMA* 1988; 260:1272–9.

Antman EM, Lau J, Kupelnick B, Mosteller F, Chalmers TC. Comparison of results of meta-analyses of randomized controlled trials and recommendations of clinical experts. *JAMA* 1992; 268:240–8.

Ashmos DP, Duchon D, McDaniel RR Jr. Organizational responses to complexity: the effect on organizational performance. *J Organ Change Manag* 2000; 13:577–94.

Atkinson M, El-Guebaly N. Research productivity among PhD faculty members and affiliates responding to the Canadian Association of Professors of Psychiatry and Canadian Psychiatric Association survey. *Can J Psychiatry* 1996; 41:509–12.

Backer P. National and international research in the future in general practice. *Scand J Prim Health Care* 1993; 11(suppl 2):4–6.

Baldwin CD, Goldblum RM, Rassin DK, Levine HG. Facilitating faculty development and research through critical review of grant proposals and articles. *Acad Med* 1994; 69:62–4.

Baldwin RG. Issues in faculty personnel policies: variety and productivity in faculty careers. *New Direct Higher Educ* 1983; 41:63–79.

Barabasi AL. *Linked*. New York: Penguin Group, 2003.

Barnett RL, Carr P, Boisnier AD *et al*. Relationships of gender and career motivation to medical faculty members' production of academic publications. *Acad Med* 1998; 73:180–6.

Barrow LH. Longitudinal study of career productivity of the most prolific science education researchers. *Educ Res Q* 2002; 25:20–7.

Bartle SA, Fink AA, Hayes BC. Psychology of the scientist. *Psychol Rep* 2000; 86:771–88.

Barton S. Chaos, self-organization, and psychology. *Am Psychol* 1994; 49:5–14.

Bar-Yam Y. Complexity rising: from human beings to human civilization, a complexity profile. In: *Encyclopedia of Life Support Systems (EOLSS)*, developed under the auspices of the UNESCO, EOLSS Publishers, Oxford, UK, 2002. http://www.eolss.net (accessed 4 October 2005). Also NECSI Technical Report 1997-12-01 (December 1997).

Bar-Yam Y. *Dynamics of Complex Systems*. Reading, MA: Perseus Books, 1997.

Bawden JW. Education research and service. *J Dental Educ* 1983; 47:289–94.

Beasley BW, Wright SM, Cofrancesco J Jr *et al.* Promotion criteria for clinician-educators in the United States and Canada. *JAMA* 1997; 278:723–8.

Beasley JW. Structure and activity of primary care research networks. *Fam Pract Res J* 1993; 13:395–403.

Beattie DS. Expanding the view of scholarship. *Acad Med* 2000; 75:871–6.

Bennett DE, Beckley PD. Surveying research interests, needs and productivity of perfusion educators. *J Extra-Corpor Technol* 1987; 19:384–91.

Blake DJ, Lezotte DC, Yablon S, Rondinelli RD. Structured research training in residency training programs. *Am J Phys Med Rehab* 1994; 73:245–50.

Bland CJ, Chou SN, Schwenk TL. Productive organization. In: J Ridky, GF Sheldon (eds). *Managing in Academics*. St. Louis: Quality Medical Publishing, 1993, pp. 26–60.

Bland CJ, Ridky J. Human and organizational resource development. In: J Ridky, GF Sheldon (eds). *Managing in Academics*. St. Louis: Quality Medical Publishing, 1993, pp. 130–58.

Bland CJ, Ruffin MT IV. Characteristics of a productive research environment. *Acad Med* 1992; 67:385–97.

Bland CJ, Schmitz CC. Characteristics of the successful researcher and implications for faculty development. *J Med Educ* 1986; 61:22–31.

Bland CJ, Weber-Main AM, Lund SM, Finstad DA. *Research-Productive Department*. Boston: Anker Publishing Company, Inc., 2005.

Bland CJ, Wersal L, Van Loy W, Jacott W. Evaluating faculty performance. *Acad Med* 2002; 77:15–30.

Block SD, Clark-Chiarelli N, Peters AS, Singer JD. Academia's chilly climate for primary care. *JAMA* 1996; 276:677–82.

Bogdewic S. Advancement and promotion: managing the individual career. In: WC McGaghie and JJ Frey. *Handbook for Academic Physicians*. New York: Springer-Verlag, 1986, pp. 22–36.

Bower DJ, Diehr S, Morzinski JA, Simpson DE. Support-challenge-vision. *Med Teacher* 1998; 20:545–7.

Bowman MA, Haynes RA, Rivo ML, Killian CD, Davis H. Characteristics of medical students by level of interest in family practice. *Fam Med* 1996; 28:713–19.

Brancati FL, Mead LA, Levine DM, Martin D, Margolis S, Klag MJ. Early predictors of career achievement in academic medicine. *JAMA* 1992; 267:1372–6.

Brocato JJ, Mavis B. Research productivity of faculty in family medicine departments at U.S. medical schools. *Acad Med* 2005; 80:244–52.

Brock WA, Hsieh DA, LeBaron B. *Non-linear Dynamics, Chaos, and Instability*. Cambridge, MA: MIT Press, 1991.

Brotherton SE, Tang SS, O'Connor KG. Trends in practice characteristics. *Pediatrics* 1997; 100:8–18.

Campbell EG, Weissman JS, Moy E, Blumenthal D. Status of clinical research in academic health centers. *JAMA* 2001; 286:800–6.

Campbell JD, Longo DL. Building research capacity in family medicine. *J Fam Pract* 2002; 51:593.

Campos-Outcalt D, Senf J. Family medicine research funding. *Fam Med* 1999; 31:709–12.

Cebul RD. Randomized, controlled trials using the Metro Firm System. *Med Care* 1991; 29(7 suppl):JS9–18.

Cheng Y, van de Ven AH. Learning the innovation journey. *Organization Sci* 1996; 7:593–614.

Christini D, Collins J, Linsay P. Experimental control of high dimensional chaos. *Phys Rev E* 1996; 54:4824–7.

Clickner DA, Martin MA, Newton M, Yablon DH. Nursing research conferences. *J NY State Nurses Assoc* 1998; 29:9–12.

Cohen NH. *Mentoring Adult Learners: a guide for educators and trainers*. Melbourne, FL: Krieger Publishing Company, 1995.

Collins BA. Review and integration of knowledge about faculty research productivity. *J Prof Nurs* 1993; 9:159–68.

Colton MR. Research: will it help us come to age as a profession? *J Nurs Leadership Manage* 1980; December:12–14.

Connelly DP, Rich EC, Curley SP, Kelly JT. Knowledge resource preferences of family physicians. *J Fam Pract* 1990; 30:353–9.

Cooper GS, Zangwill L. Analysis of the quality of research reports in the *Journal of General Internal Medicine*. *J Gen Intern Med* 1989; 4:232–6.

Copp LA. Deans identify factors which inhibit and facilitate nursing research. *J Adv Nurs* 1984; 9:513–17.

Covey SR. *Seven Habits Of Highly Effective People*. New York: Simon and Schuster, 1989.

Culpepper L, Franks P. Family medicine research. *JAMA* 1983; 249:63–8.

Curry L, MacIntyre K. Content of family practice. *Can Fam Physician* 1982; 28:124–6.

Curtis P. What kind of research in family medicine – further reflections. *Fam Med Teacher* 1980; 12:8–11.

Curtis P, Dickinson P, Steiner J, Lanphear B, Vu K. Building capacity for research in family medicine. *Fam Med* 2003; 35:124–30.

Curtis P, Reid A, Newton W. Primary care research fellowship. *Fam Med* 1992; 24:586–90.

Curtis P, Shaffer VD, Goldstein AO, Seufert L. Counting the cost of an NRSA primary care research fellowship program. *Fam Med* 1998; 30:17–21.

Davies HD, Langley JM, Speert DP. Rating authors' contribution to collaborative research. *Can Med Assoc J* 1996; 155:877–82.

DeHaven MJ, Wilson GR, Murphee DD. Developing a research program in a community-based department of family medicine. *Fam Med* 1994; 26:303–8.

DeHaven MJ, Wilson GR, Murphee DD, Grundig JP. Family practice residency program directors' views on research. *Fam Med* 1997; 29:33–7.

DeHaven MJ, Wilson GR, O'Connor-Kettlestrings P. Creating a research culture. *Fam Med* 1998; 30:501–7.

Dendrinos D, Sonis M. *Chaos and Socio-Spacial Dynamics*. NY: Springer-Verlag, 1990.

Dickinson WP, Stange KC, Ebell MH, Ewigman BG, Green LA. Involving all family physicians and family medicine faculty members in the use and generation of new knowledge. *Fam Med* 2000; 32:480–90.

Dooley K. Complex adaptive systems model of organizational change. *Non-linear Dynamics Psychol Life Sci* 1997; 1:69–97.

Dooley K, Johnson T, Bush D. TQM, chaos, and complexity. *Human Syst Manage* 1995; 14:1–16.

Ebell MH, Barry HC, Slawson DC, Shaughnessy AF. Finding POEMs in the medical literature. *J Fam Pract* 1999; 48:350–5.

Eisenberg JM. Cultivating a new field. *J Gen Intern Med* 1986; 1(suppl):S8–S18.

Eisenhardt KM. Speed and strategic choice: How managers accelerate decision making. *Calif Manage Rev* 1990; 2:39–54.

Elder NC, Blake RL Jr. Publication patterns of presentations at the Society of Teachers of Family Medicine and North American Primary Care Research Group annual meetings. *Fam Med* 1994; 26:352–5.

El-Guebaly N, Atkinson M. Research training and productivity among faculty. *Can J Psychiatry* 1996; 41:144–9.

Elward KS, Goldstein AO, Ruffin MT. Fellowship training in family medicine. *Fam Med* 1994; 26:376–81.

Emanuel EJ, Wendler D, Grady C. What makes clinical research ethical? *JAMA* 2000; 283:2701–11.

Fairweather JS. Mythologies of faculty productivity. *J Higher Educ* 2002; 73:26–48.

Fang D, May E, Colburn L, Hurley J. Racial and ethnic disparities in faculty promotion in academic medicine. *JAMA* 2000; 284:1085–92.

Ferrer R, Katerndahl D. Predictors of short-term and long-term scholarly activity by academic faculty. *Fam Med* 2002; 34:455–61.

Flexner A. *Medical Education in the United States and Canada*. NY: Carnegie Foundation for the Advancement of Teaching, 1910.

Flocke SA, Zyzanski SJ, Pomiecko G. Prospective study of medical faculty promotion and tenure. Personal communication, 2004.

Freeman W. Physiology of perception. *Sci Am* 1991; 264(February):78–85.

Frey JJ, Frey J. Literature analysis in family medicine and general practice. *Fam Med* 1981; 13:7–10.

Fried LP, Francomano CA, MacDonald SM *et al.* Career development for women in academic medicine. *JAMA* 1996; 276:898–905.

Future of Family Medicine Project Leadership Committee. Future of family medicine. *Ann Fam Med* 2004; 2(suppl 1):S3–S32.

Geyman JP. Research in the family practice residency program. *J Fam Pract* 1977; 5:245–8.

Geyman JP. Climate for research in family practice. *J Fam Pract* 1978; 7:69–74.

Geyman JP, Berg AO. *Journal of Family Practice*, 1974–1983. *J Fam Pract* 1984; 18:47–51.

Geyman JP, Berg AO. *Journal of Family Practice*, 1974–1988. *J Fam Pract* 1989; 28:301–4.

Gilchrist V, Miller RS, Gillanders WR *et al.* Does family practice at residency teaching sites reflect community practice? *J Fam Pract* 1993; 37:555–63.

Gjerde C. Where are articles by candidates for academic promotion published? *J Fam Pract* 1992; 34:449–53.

Gjerde C. Faculty promotion and publication rates in family medicine. *Fam Med* 1994; 26:361–5.

Gjerde C, Clements W, Clements B. Publication characteristics of family practice faculty nominated for academic promotion. *J Fam Pract* 1982; 15:663–6.

Goldberger AL, Rigney DR, Mietus J, Antman EM, Greenwald S. Non-linear dynamics in sudden cardiac death syndrome. *Experientia* 1988; 44:983–7.

Goldberger AL, West BJ. Applications of non-linear dynamics to clinical cardiology. *Ann NY Acad Sci* 1987; 504:195–211.

Goldman L. Blueprint for a research career in general internal medicine. *J Gen Intern Med* 1991; 6:341–4.

Gonzales AO, Westfall J, Barley GE. Promoting medical student involvement in primary care research. *Fam Med* 1998; 30:113–16.

Gorman PN, Helfand M. Information seeking in primary care. *Med Decis Making* 1995; 15:113–19.

Grams KM, Christ MA. Faculty workload formulas in nursing education. *J Prof Nurs* 1992; 8:96–104.

Green LA, Fryer GE. Development and goals of the AAFP Center for Policy Studies in Family Practice and Primary Care. *J Fam Pract* 1999; 48:905–8.

Green LA, Lutz LJ. Notions about networks. In: J Mayfield, ML Grady (eds). *Primary Care Research*. Washington, DC: U.S. DHHS, PHS, AHCPR, 1990, pp. 125–32.

Green LA, Niebauer LJ, Miller RS, Lutz LJ. Analysis of reasons for discontinuing participation in a practice-based research network. *Fam Med* 1991; 23:447–9.

Green LA, Wood M, Becker L *et al.* Ambulatory sentinel practice network. *J Fam Pract* 1984; 18:275–80.

Grzybowski SCW, Bates J, Calam B *et al.* Physician peer support writing group. *Fam Med* 2003; 35:195–201.

Guastello S. *Chaos, Catastrophe, and Human Affairs*. Mahwah, NJ: Erlbaum, 1995.

Harris DL, DaRosa DA, Liu PL, Hash RB. Facilitating academic institutional change. *Fam Med* 2003; 35:187–94.

Haynes RB, McKibbon KA, Fitzgerald D *et al.* How to keep up with the medical literature: why try to keep up and how to get started. *Ann Intern Med* 1986; 105:149–53.

Healy B. Innovators for the 21st century. *N Engl J Med* 1988; 319:1058–64.

Hekelman FP, Gilchrist V, Zyzanski SJ, Glover P, Olness K. Educational intervention to increase faculty publication productivity. *Fam Med* 1995a; 27:255–9.

Hekelman FP, Zyzanski SJ, Flocke SA. Successful and less-successful research performance of junior faculty. *Res Higher Educ* 1995b; 36:235–55.

Hitchcock MA, Bland CJ, Hekelman FP, Blumenthal MG. Professional networks. *Acad Med* 1995; 70:1108–16.

Holland JH. *Hidden Order.* Reading, MA: Addison-Wesley Publishing Company, 1995.

Hollenberg CH. Nurturing the young academician. *Clin Invest Med* 1992; 15:252–4.

Holloway RL, Bland CJ. Academic freedom and family medicine. *Fam Med* 1984; 16:225–6.

Holloway RL, Bland CJ, Schmitz CC, Withington AM. Advanced research seminar series for family medicine faculty members. *Fam Med* 1988; 20:338–42.

Hueston WJ. Comparison of university and community-based family practice physician educators. *Fam Med* 1993a; 25:576–9.

Hueston WJ. Factors associated with research efforts of academic family physicians. *J Fam Pract* 1993b; 37:44–8.

Hueston WJ, Mainous AG. Family medicine research in the community setting. *J Fam Pract* 1996; 43:171–6.

Huth EJ. Primary care research environment. *J Gen Intern Med* 1986; 1(suppl):s1–s7.

Ingram TG. Cross-sectional analysis of family medicine publications in the indexed medical literature. *Fam Med* 1992; 24:303–6.

Institute of Medicine. *Primary Care: America's health in a new era.* Washington, DC: Institute of Medicine, 1996.

Irvine AA, Phillips EK, Fisher M, Cloonan P. Out of the ivory tower. *Home Health Care Serv Quart* 1990; 10:117–30.

Jaen CR, Stange KC, Nutting PA. Competing demands of primary care. *J Fam Pract* 1994; 38:166–71.

Jones RF, Gold JS. Faculty appointment and tenure policies in medical schools. *Acad Med* 1998; 73:211–19.

Jungnickel PW, Creswell JW. Workplace correlates and scholarly performance of clinical pharmacy faculty. *EDRS Microfiche*, ED 352916, 1992.

Katerndahl DA. Factors chosen by departmental chairs as important to family medicine. *Fam Pract Res J* 1994; 14:177–81.

Katerndahl DA. *Predictive Validity of an Instrument to Assess Success in Medical Researchers.* Presented at the North American Primary Care Research Group meeting, November 8–11, 1995, Houston, Texas.

Katerndahl DA. Associations between departmental features and departmental scholarly activity. *Fam Med* 1996; 28:119–27.

Katerndahl DA. Effect of attendance at an annual primary care research methods conference on research productivity and development. *Fam Med* 2000a; 32:701–8.

Katerndahl DA. Preliminary Evidence for Modeling Departmental Scholarly Productivity as a *Complex Adaptive System.* Presented at North American Primary Care Research Group, November 4–7, 2000b, Amelia Island, Florida.

Katerndahl D. Lifetime of touching patients' lives (editorial). *Fam Med* 2003; 35:365–6.

Katerndahl DA, Burge SK, Schneider FD, Legler J. Clinical content of the family practice research literature. *Texas Fam Phys* 1998; July/August:26–7.

Katerndahl DA, McDaniel RR Jr. *Dynamic Patterns of Scholarly Productivity among Faculty with Low, Moderate, and High Productivity.* Presentation at annual meeting of North American Primary Care Research Group, October 25–28, 2003, Banff, Alberta.

Katerndahl DA, McDaniel RR Jr. *Building Research Capacity Based on Dynamic Patterns of*

Scholarly Activity. Workshop presentation at annual conference of North American Primary Care Research Group, October 10–13, 2004, Orlando, Florida.

Katerndahl D, Parchman M, Larme A. Cultural (R)evolution (editorial). *Fam Med* 2002; 34:616–18.

Katz JN, Solomon DH, Bates DW. Differences between generalists and specialists (editorial). *Arthritis Care Res* 1997; 10:161–2.

Kauffman SA. *Origins of Order*. New York: Oxford University Press, 1993.

Kazerooni E. Introduction to academic radiology. *Acad Radiol* 1997; 4:390–7.

Kenkre JE, Hobbs FDR, Greenfield SM. Research activity in general practice (letter). *Br J Gen Pract* 1993; 43:535.

Kohlenberg EM. Faculty research productivity and organizational structure in schools of nursing. *J Prof Nurs* 1992; 8:271–5.

Korenman SG, Berk R, Wenger NS, Lew V. Evaluation of the research norms of scientists and administrators responsible for academic research integrity. *JAMA* 1998; 279:41–7.

Kuzel AJ, Piotrowski ZH. Family practice resident research in Illinois. *Fam Med* 1984; 16:3–6.

Liebovitch LS. *Fractals and Chaos*. New York: Oxford University Press, 1998.

Luis Palau Evangelistic Association. *Friendship Evangelism*. Portland, OR: Luis Palau Evangelistic Association, 1988.

Luukonen T. Bibliometrics and evaluation of research performance. *Ann Med* 1990; 22:145–50.

Mainous A. Importance of track records in developing family medicine research (editorial). *Fam Med* 2003; 35:138–40.

Mainous AG, Bowman MA, Zoller JS. Importance of interpersonal relationship factors in decisions regarding authorship. *Fam Med* 2002; 34:462–7.

Mainous AG, Hueston WJ, Ye X, Bazell C. Comparison of family medicine research in research intense and less intense institutions. *Arch Fam Med* 2000; 9:1100–4.

Marchiori DM, Meeker W, Hawk C, Long CR. Research productivity of chiropractic college faculty. *J Manipulative Physiol Therapeutics* 1998; 21:8–13.

Martin BR, Irvine J. Assessing basic research. *Res Policy* 1983; 12:61–90.

Marvel MK, Staehling S, Hendricks B. Taxonomy of clinical research methods. *Fam Med* 1991; 23:202–7.

May JJ. Policy uses of research. *Inquiry* 1975; 12:228–30.

McDaniel RR Jr, Driebe DJ. Complexity science and health care management. In: JD Blair, MD Fottler, G Savage (eds). *Advances in Health Care Management* Vol. 2. Stamford, CN: JAI Press, 2001, pp. 11–36.

McDaniel RR Jr, Jordan ME, Fleeman BF. Surprise, surprise, surprise! A complexity science view of the unexpected. *Health Care Manage Rev* 2003; 28:266–78.

McKinley W, Cheng JLC, Schick AG. Perceptions of resource criticality in times of resource scarcity. *Acad Manage J* 1986; 29:623–32.

McNeely JB, Moody LE, Anderson GC. Endowed research chairs. *J Prof Nurs* 1987; 3:114–17.

McWhinney IR. General practice as an academic discipline. *Lancet* 1966; February 19:419–23.

Megel ME, Langston NF, Creswell JW. Scholarly productivity. *J Prof Nurs* 1988; 4:45–54.

Merenstein J, Rao G, D'Amico F. Clinical research in family medicine. *Fam Med* 2003; 35:284–8.

Miller MD. Ratings of medical journals by family physician educators. *J Fam Pract* 1982; 15:517–19.

Miller WL, Crabtree BF, McDaniel R, Stange KC. Understanding change in primary care practice using complexity theory. *J Fam Pract* 1998; 46:369–76.

Mills OF, Zyzanski SJ, Flocke S. Factors associated with research productivity in family practice residencies. *Fam Med* 1995; 27:188–93.

Morahan P. How to establish and support formal mentoring programs. *Acad Physician Scientist* 2001; January–February:8.

Morel B, Ramanujam R. Through the looking glass of complexity: the dynamics of organizations as adaptive and evolving systems. *Organ Sci* 1999; 10:278–93.

Morrison F. *Art of Modeling Dynamic Systems*. New York: Wiley, 1991.

Morzinski JA. Influence of academic projects on the professional socialization of family medicine faculty. *Fam Med* 2005; 37:348–53.

Morzinski JA, Simpson DE. Outcomes of a comprehensive faculty development program for local, full-time faculty. *Fam Med* 2003; 25:434–9.

Morzinski JA, Simpson DE, Bower DJ, Diehr S. Faculty development through formal mentoring. *Acad Med* 1994; 69:267–9.

Mukamal KJ, Smetana GW, Delbanco T. Clinicians, educators, and investigators in general internal medicine. *J Gen Intern Med* 2002; 17:565–71.

Mularski CA, Bradigan PS. Academic health sciences librarians' publication patterns. *Bull Med Libr Assoc* 1991; 79:168–77.

Muncie HL Jr, Sobal J, DeForge BR. NAPCRG abstracts 1977–1987. *Fam Med* 1990; 22:125–9.

Mundt MH. External mentor program. *J Prof Nurs* 2001; 17(1):40–5.

Murata PJ, Lynch WD, Puffer JC, Green LA. Attitudes toward and experience in research among family medicine chairs. *J Fam Pract* 1992; 35:417–21.

NAPCRG Committee on Building Research Capacity, Academic Family Medicine Organizations Research Subcommittee. What does it mean to build research capacity? *Fam Med* 2002; 34:678–84.

National Institutes of Health (NIH). *2001 Extramural Awards Ranking Tables*. Rockville, MD: NIH, Office of Extramural Research, 2002.

Neale AV. National survey of research requirements for family practice residents and faculty. *Fam Med* 2002; 34:262–7.

Newman MEJ. Structure of scientific collaboration networks. *Proc Natl Acad Sci* 2001; 98:404–9.

Newman MEJ. Coauthorship networks and patterns of scientific collaboration. *Proc Natl Acad Sci* 2004; 101(suppl 1):5200–5.

Oeffinger KC, Roaten SP Jr, Ader DN, Buchanan RJ. Support and rewards for scholarly activity in family medicine. *Fam Med* 1997; 29:508–12.

Oinonen MJ, Crowley WF Jr, Moskowitz J, Vlasses PH. How do academic health centers value and encourage clinical research? *Acad Med* 2001; 76:700–6.

Osborn EHS, Pettiti DB. Physician interest in collaborative research. *J Am Board Fam Pract* 1988; 1:29–32.

Overman ES. New science of management. *J Public Adm Res Theory* 1996; 6:75–89.

Page IH. Research – its many forms and nurture. *Biosci Commun* 1976; 2:56–64.

Palepu A, Friedman RH, Barnett RC *et al*. Junior faculty members' mentoring relationships and their professional development in U.S. medical schools. *Acad Med* 1998; 73:318–23.

Parchman M, Katerndahl D, Larme A. Family medicine and research: from here to eternity (editorial). *Fam Med* 2003; 35:345–9.

Parkerson GR Jr, Barr DM, Bass M *et al*. Meeting the challenge of research in family medicine. *J Fam Pract* 1982; 14:105–13.

Paterson M, Baker D, Gable C, Michael S, Wintch K. Faculty research productivity in allied health settings. *J Allied Health* 1993; Summer issue:249–61.

Pathman D, Gamble G, Samruddhi T, Newton W. *Report on Research Productivity in Family Medicine*. Kansas City: NAPCRG, 2002.

Pathman D, Viera A, Newton W. *Building Family Medicine Research in the U.S.* Workshop presentation at annual conference of North American Primary Care Research Group, October 15–18, 2005, Quebec City, Quebec.

Perkoff GT. Research in family medicine. *J Fam Pract* 1981; 13:553–7.

Perkoff GT. Research environment in family practice. *J Fam Pract* 1985; 5:389–93.

Perkoff GT. To be a mentor. *Fam Med* 1992; 24:584–5.

Peterson M, Baker D, Gable C, Michael S, Wintch K. Faculty research productivity in allied health settings. *J Allied Health* 1993; Summer:249–61.

Pitts J. General practice research in the Journal (letter). *Br J Gen Pract* 1991; 41(342):34–5.

Prescott K, Lloyd M, Douglas HR *et al*. Promoting clinically effective practice. *Fam Pract* 1997; 14:320–3.

Price DJP. *Little Science, Big Science*. NY: Columbia University Press, 1963.

Prochaska JO, DiClemente CC. Toward a comprehensive model of change. In: WR Miller, N Heather (eds). *Treating Addictive Behaviors*. New York: Plenum Press, 1986, pp. 3–27.

Ragins BR, Cotton JL. Gender and willingness to mentor in organizations. *J Manage* 1993; 19:97–111.

Rajan TV, Clive J. NIH research grants (letter). *JAMA* 2000; 283:1963.

Ramos K, Unscheid R, Schafer S. Real-time information-seeking behavior of residency physicians. *Fam Med* 2003; 35:257–60.

Ramos-Remus C, Orozco-Barocio G, Suarez-Almazor M *et al*. Research in rheumatology. *Clin Exp Rheumatol* 1993; 11:71–4.

Reid A, Stritter FT, Arndt JE. Assessment of faculty development program outcomes. *Fam Med* 1997; 29:242–7.

Rhoades G. Managing productivity in an academic institution. *Res Higher Educ* 2001; 42:619–32.

Richards JG. General practice research in New Zealand. *J Fam Pract* 1980; 10:1097–9.

Rodnick JE. Research fellowships (editorial). *Fam Med* 1999; 31:438–9.

Rogers JC, Holloway RL, Miller SM. Academic mentoring and family medicine's research productivity. *Fam Med* 1990; 22:186–90.

Rothman J, Badyrka R. Entry-level research. *Clin Manage* 1991; 11:38–41.

Ruffin MT, Sheets KJ. Primary care research funding sources. *J Fam Pract* 1992; 35:281–7.

Sands RG, Parson LA, Duane J. Faculty mentoring faculty in a public university. *J Higher Educ* 1991; 62:174–92.

Schaad DC, Byers PH, Davidson RC *et al*. Relation of students' premedical majors to participation in research in medical school. *J Med Educ* 1984; 59:54–7.

Scheid DC, Hamm RM, Crawford SA. Measuring academic production. *Fam Med* 2002; 34:34–44.

Scheid D, Logue E, Gilchrist VJ *et al*. Do we practice what we preach? *Fam Med* 1995; 27:519–24.

Scherger JE, Young HF. AAFP research initiative (editorial). *J Fam Pract* 1998; 46:203–4.

Schwartz K, Northrup J, Israel N *et al*. Use of on-line evidence-based resources at the point of care. *Fam Med* 2003; 35:251–6.

Senge PM. *The Fifth Discipline*. NY: Currency Doubleday, 1990.

Shapiro J, Coggen P, Rubel A *et al*. Process of faculty-mentored student research in family medicine. *Fam Med* 1994; 26:283–9.

Sharp LF, Priesmeyer HR. Tutorial: chaos theory. *Qual Manage Health Care* 1995; 3:71–86.

Silagy CA, Jewell D. Review of 39 years of randomized controlled trials in the *British Journal of General Practice*. *Br J Gen Pract* 1994; 44:359–63.

Silagy CA, Jewell D, Mant D. Analysis of randomized controlled trials published in the U.S. family medicine literature, 1987–1991. *J Fam Pract* 1994; 39:236–42.

Silagy CA, Schattner P, Baxter RG. Current status of general practice research in Australia. *Med J Australia* 1992; 157:108–13.

Slatkoff SF, Curtis P, Coker A. Patients as subjects for research. *J Am Board Fam Pract* 1994; 7:196–201.

Smith BWH. Chaotic family dynamics. *Arch Fam Med* 1994; 3:231–8.

Sonis J, Joines J. Quality of clinical trials published in the *Journal of Family Practice* 1974–1991. *J Fam Pract* 1994; 39:225–35.

Stange KC. Primary care research: barriers and opportunities. *J Fam Pract* 1996; 42:192–8.

Stange KC, Hekelman FP. Mentoring needs and family medicine faculty. *Fam Med* 1990; 22:183–5.

Stange KC, Miller WL, McWhinney I. Developing the knowledge base of family practice. *Fam Med* 2001; 33:286–97.

Taniguchi MH, Johnson PD. Rehabilitation resident academic productivity. *Am J Phys Med Rehab* 1994; 73:240–4.

Taylor RB. View to the future of family practice. *Med Times* 1990; 118:31–5.

Taylor RB, Colwill JM, Puffer JC *et al*. Success strategies for departments of family medicine. *J Am Board Fam Pract* 1991; 4:427–36.

Taylor JS, Friedman RH, Speckman JL *et al*. Fellowship training and career outcomes for primary care physician-faculty. *Acad Med* 2001; 76:366–72.

Temte JL, Hunter PH, Beasley JW. Factors associated with research interest and activity during family practice residency. *Fam Med* 1994; 26:93–7.

Verhoeven AAH, Boerma EJ, Meyboom-de Jong B. Use of information sources by family physicians. *Bull Med Libr Assoc* 1995; 83:85–90.

Vieira D, Faraino R. Analyzing the research record of an institution's list of faculty publications. *Bull Med Libr Assoc* 1997; 85:154–7.

Virginia Commonwealth University. *Faculty Mentoring Guide*. Richmond: Virginia Commonwealth University, 1997.

Vydareny KH, Waldrop SM, Jackson VP *et al*. Road to success. *Acad Radiol* 1999; 6:564–9.

Vydareny KH, Waldrop SM, Jackson VP *et al*. Career advancement of men and women in academic radiology. *Acad Radiol* 2000; 7:493–501.

Wagner PJ, Hornsby JL, Talbert FS *et al*. Publication productivity in academic family medicine departments. *Fam Med* 1994; 26:366–9.

Wakefield-Fisher M. Relationship between professionalization of nursing faculty, leadership styles of deans, and faculty scholarly productivity. *J Prof Nurs* 1987; 3:155–64.

Wallace DP. Most productive faculty. *Library J* 1990; 115:61–3.

Waller KV, Wyatt D, Karni KR. Scholarly activities among clinical laboratory science faculty. *Clin Lab Sci* 1999; 12:19–27.

Watson PG. Faculty research skills development. *J Allied Health* 1990; Winter:25–37.

Weick KE. *Sensemaking in Organizations*. Thousand Oaks, CA: SAGE Publications, Inc, 1995.

Weiss BD. Publications by family physicians in non-family medicine journals. *Fam Pract Res J* 1990; 10:117–22.

Weiss BD. Why family practice research? (editorial). *Arch Fam Med* 2000; 9:1105–7.

Weiss BD. Publications by family medicine faculty in the biomedical literature: 1989–1999. *Fam Med* 2002; 34:10–16.

Weissman JS, Saglam D, Campbell EG, Causino N, Blumenthal D. Market forces and unsponsored research in academic health centers. *JAMA* 1999; 281:1093–8.

West BJ, Goldberger AL, Rovner G, Bhargava V. Non-linear dynamics of the heartbeat. *Physica* 1985; 17D:198–206.

Wilson JL, Redman RW. Research policies and practices in family practice residencies. *J Fam Pract* 1980; 10:479–83.

Yeragani VK, Jampala VC, Sobelewski E, Kay J, Igel G. Effects of paroxetine on heart period variability in patients with panic disorder. *Neuropsychobiology* 1999; 40:124–8.

Yip CC, Waxman R. 10-year (1986–1995) review of data on scholar awardees in faculty of medicine, University of Toronto. *Clin Invest Med* 1997; 20:280–2.

Zarin DA, Pincus HA, West JC, McIntyre JS. Practice-based research in psychiatry. *Am J Psychiatry* 1997; 154:1199–208.

Zyzanski SJ, Williams RL, Flocke SA, Acheson LS, Kelly RB. Academic achievement of successful candidates for tenure and promotion to associate professor. *Fam Med* 1996; 28:358–63.

Career Development

Questions to Answer

Job

1. Why are you in your current position?
2. What is your job description?
3. What is your position as related to departmental needs?
4. How do you spend your professional time?

Career Opportunities

5. What are your career goals?
6. How will you evaluate whether you are meeting your goals?

Growth Opportunities

7. What do you need for personal growth?
8. Are you receiving adequate support?
9. Is this a productive work environment?

Long-Term Career Goals Instrument

For each of the five areas below, indicate what career goal(s) you have and by when you hope to achieve them. (List more than one goal per area if appropriate.)

Area	Career Goal(s)	Achieved by?
Focus for Your Research[a]		
Administrative Position(s)[b]		
Promotion/Tenure[c]		
National Reputation[d]		
Grants[e]		

[a] e.g. "Track record in doctor-patient relationship research."
[b] e.g. "Become department chair."
[c] e.g. "Promoted to full professor," "Tenured."
[d] e.g. "Accepted as authority on my focus by national organizations."
[e] e.g. "Received R01 grant."

Job Activity Analysis Instrument

(Adapted from Bogdewic, 1986)

Directions: List your key activities and the amount (%) of time you devote to them. Then rate the value of each activity to the program and to you, as well as your level of satisfaction.

Key Activities	% of Your Time for This Activity	Value of This Activity to the Program?	Value of This Activity to You?	Your Level of Satisfaction?
1.				
2.				
3.				
4.				
5.				

Survey of Scholarly Activity Instrument

Please complete the following related to your activities during the previous year.

1. Indicate the current status of all RESEARCH studies in which you have been involved.

Study Title	List Co-investigators	Are You Principal Investigator on the Study?	Current Status																		
			In Progress									Completed				Submitted, Not Accepted		Accepted	
			Planning	Design	Select/Develop Instruments	IRB Approval	Pilot Study	Funding	Sample Identification	Data Collection	Data Analysis	Interpretation of Results	No of Manuscripts	Manuscripts in Preparation	Completed	Publication[a]	Presentation[b]	Publication[c]	Presentation[d]

[a] Specify number of times it has been submitted.
[b] Please indicate number of times it has been presented outside of your institution.
[c] Specify journal names.
[d] Specify conference names.

2. Indicate the current status of all NON-RESEARCH scholarly activity.

Project Title	List Co-authors	Are You Principal Investigator?	In Preparation	Submitted, Not Accepted		Accepted	
				Publication[a]	Presentation[b]	Publication[c]	Presentation[d]

[a] Specify number of times it has been submitted.
[b] Please indicate number of times it has been presented outside of your institution.
[c] Specify journal names.
[d] Specify conference names.

3. Please indicate all new grants in which you participated (do not include continuation grants).

Title	Grant Agency	Co-investigator(s)	Were You Principal Investigator?	Current Status	Is This a Research Grant?	Dollar Amount	
						Total Direct Cost	Direct Costs Going to Department

F = Funded.
A = Approved but not Funded.
I = Pending.
R = Rejected.

Your Current Status Instrument

Collaborators

With whom do you currently collaborate on research and what is their expertise?

Within Department		Within Institution		Outside Institution	
Name	Expertise	Name	Expertise	Name	Expertise

With whom would you like to collaborate on research in the future?

Mentors

List individuals that you consider to be your mentor and in what area(s) they mentor you.

Within Department		Within Institution		Outside Institution	
Name	Area Mentored[a]	Name	Area Mentored	Name	Area Mentored

[a] i. e. Professional socialization, role model, nurturing, teaching, advocacy.

List individuals who are not currently your mentor but with whom you would like to have a mentor relationship.

Institutional Resources and Opportunities Instrument

Possible Collaborators

Please list names of all of the possible collaborators *not* currently used by you within your department and institution in each of four areas.

Area	Department	Institution
Research Focus		
Methodology		
Statistics		
Grantsmanship		

Possible Mentors

Please list names of all of the possible mentors *not* currently used by you within your department and institution in each of five areas.

Area	Department	Institution
Professional Socialization		
Role Model		
Nurturing		
Teaching		
Advocacy		

Fellowship/Advanced Training or Degrees

Please list names all known opportunities for advanced training (fellowships; MS, MPH, and PhD degrees; courses; conferences) within your department, institution, community, and state.

Department		Institution		Community		State	
Activity	Time Commitment	Activity	Time Commitment	Activity	Time Commitment	Activity	Time Commitment

Institutional Facilities

Indicate if your institution has the following facilities and the level of support that they will provide to faculty members.

Facility	Available?	Level of Support
Extensive Library		
Computing Resources		
Statistical Services		
Office of Instructional Development		
Institutional Review Board		
Grants Management Office		
Promotion and Tenure Committee		
Other: _____		

Departmental Resources

Indicate which resources are available in your department.

Resources	Available?
Clerical Assistants	
Statistician	
Research Assistants	
Computer Support	
Internet Access	
Departmental Library	
Interlibrary Loans	
Scientific Writer	
Grant Writer	
Travel Funds for Conferences	
Fund for Pilot Studies	

Departmental and Institutional Opportunities

List all known opportunities that are available and describe them.

Opportunity	Department	Institution
Faculty Development		
Faculty Awards		
Faculty Evaluation and Feedback		

Departmental Resources Development Activities

List all faculty development activities available in your department.

Activity	Available?
Faculty Development Seminars	
Teaching Skills	
Research Skills	
Computer Skills	
Writing Skills	
Grantsmanship Skills	
Administrative Skills	
Review of Draft Manuscripts	
Review of Grant Proposals	
Review of Research Study Ideas	
Annual Promotion and Tenure Review	
Annual Review with Chair	

Availability of Grant Support

List all known available research grant support offered through institutional, community, and state organizations and indicate what areas of research each organization supports.

Institution		Community		State	
Grant	Area	Foundations	Areas	Foundations	Areas

Faculty Activities and Research Environment Survey (Abridged)

(Adapted from Hekelman *et al*, 1995b)

Put an "X" through responses that apply to each question. (Check only responses that apply.)

	Local Mentoring	Research Activity	Networking	Scholarly Habits
1. Do you have a focused area of research?				Yes
2. Does your department provide senior guidance in developing grant proposals?	Yes			
3. Do you have an experienced researcher *off-campus* to critique your papers or grants before submission?			Yes	
4. How do you find professional contacts?				
a. Mentors/colleagues at your institution?	Yes			
b. Mentors/colleagues outside your institution?			Yes	
5. Is there a key senior person(s) on campus who assists you in:				
a. Participating in research projects?	Yes			
b. Writing grants?	Yes			
c. Writing publications?	Yes			
d. Giving advice?	Yes			
e. Introduction to other researchers?	Yes			
6. In an average month, how many *colleagues* do you contact at your institution regarding research?		$\geqslant 3$		

Faculty Activities and Research Environment Survey (Abridged) (cont.)

7. In an average month, how many *colleagues* do you contact outside your institution regarding research?	$\geqslant 1$	$\geqslant 2$
8. In an average month, how many *times* do you contact colleagues at your institution regarding research?	$\geqslant 1$	
9. In an average month, how many *times* do you contact colleagues outside your institution regarding research?		$\geqslant 1$
10. To what degree is your department chairperson supportive of your research activities?	Above average	
11. What percentage of the members of your department would you consider to be "productive researchers"?	$> 25\%$	
12. How much do you enjoy doing research or publishing?	Very much	
13. To what degree are you abreast of the current literature in your area?		Reasonably up-to-date
14. How many formal (e.g., semester length) postgraduate courses have you had in research?		$\geqslant 5$
15. How many research workshops (1–5 days) have you attended in the last 2 years?		$\geqslant 1$
16. How many books on research have you read in the last year?		$\geqslant 1$
17. In the last 2 years, on how many grants have you been principal investigator?	$\geqslant 1$	
18. With how many different departments do you collaborate on research?	$\geqslant 2$	
19. How many research interest groups do you participate in locally?	$\geqslant 2$	
20. How many publications are you working on right now?		$\geqslant 3$

21. How many annual research meetings do you attend?				≥2
22. How many research papers did you present during the last 2 years?				≥2
23. How many of those papers were presented at national meetings?				≥2
24. What percentage of a 40-hour week does your department expect you to give to research activities?		≥25%		
Column "X" Totals Total Possible	7	9	5	8

"Research Activity" + "Scholarly Habits" = _____

25. In the last 2 years, on how many funded federal or foundation grants have you worked?		≥1
26. How many peer-reviewed publications have you had in the last 2 years?		≥4
	TOTAL "X's"	

Complexity Science Glossary

Attractors	Constructs that dictate the range of possible behaviors of a system and prevent random activity. The presence of a low-dimensional attractor produces the pattern. Whereas static system attractors have a dimension of 0, and periodic systems tend to have one-dimensional attractors, chaotic attractors have a low but non-integer dimension, and are strange
Bifurcation	The property in which small changes in the system produce abrupt, oscillatory changes in its behavior
Black Noise	Randomness showing directionality over time but with sudden catastrophic shifts
Brown Noise	Randomness in which there is accumulation of random events over time
Chaotic Dynamics	Dynamics that appear random, but the possible values are limited by the system. Chaotic dynamics produce patterns that are predictable even though the path is not
Chaotic Systems	Systems that arise when there is a delay between action and consequence, and when feedback within the system varies in strength and direction. Chaotic systems are deterministic but only over the short term, and they can be recognized by the presence of a low-dimensional attractor, sensitivity to initial conditions, and bifurcations
Clustering Coefficient	Proportion of agents within groups
Co-evolution	Change within the system as the environment changes
Complex Adaptive Systems	Systems composed of multiple components that display complexity and adaptation to input. Such systems are based on the self-organization of their components and often display non-linear dynamics
Critical Systems	Systems that depend upon self-organization and display pink noise randomness. Complex inter-relationships among components produce a system in which a single event can result in a cascading effect due to the coupling of components

Emergence	Appearance of new structure or behavior as scale changes. Emergence depends upon the presence of self-organization
Fitness Landscape	Representation of how fitness would change with different changes in the system
Linear/Periodic Dynamics	Dynamics that are cyclic and produce outputs in which both path and pattern are predictable
Network Centrality	Degree of similarity between an actual network and one connected in a star pattern to a central node
Network Cohesion	Strength of connections within a network
Network Density	Proportion of all possible connections that are realized
Network Distance	Average number of steps for any two agents to reach each other in a network
Non-linearity	Output behavior of the system is not proportional to the input
Pink Noise	Randomness with anti-persistent trends, producing a pattern in which trends over time are periodically corrected and brought back to baseline. It is also known as criticality
Random Systems	Systems in which both the path and pattern are unpredictable
Scale	Different levels within a system and can apply to levels of magnification or time
Self-organization	Structure or patterns developing within an open system. Self-organized systems have several characteristics. Not only do these systems have temporal or behavioral organization, but their processes are usually coupled; alterations in one component can cause others to change. Local instabilities in the system can cause reorganization of the whole system. Although cyclic changes can occur, behavior can be non-linear, dependent upon chaotic attractors. Finally, self-organized systems can exist in multiple stable states that can change rapidly
Sensitivity to Initial Conditions	The characteristic that a small change initially can send the system on a new trajectory, drastically changing the system's subsequent performance
Static Dynamics	Dynamics are limited to a single point
White Noise	True randomness in which there is no trend over time

Index